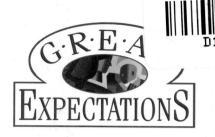

G·R·E·A·T
EXPECTATIONS

Pregnancy
Journal &
Planner

Marcie Jones & Sandy Jones
Peter S. Bernstein, MD, MPH, FACOG
Medical Consultant

Sterling Publishing, New York

Published by Sterling Publishing Co., Inc.
387 Park Avenue South, New York, NY 10016

©2005 by Marcie Jones and Sandy Jones

Distributed in Canada by Sterling Publishing
c/o Canadian Manda Group, 165 Dufferin Street
Toronto, Ontario M6K 3H6

Distributed in Great Britain by Chrysalis Books
64 Brewery Road, London N7 9NT, England

Distributed in Australia by Capricorn Link (Australia) Pty. Ltd.
P.O. Box 704, Windsor, NSW 2756, Australia

ISBN 1-4027-2824-7

Printed in Thailand by Sirivitana Interprint Public Company Ltd.

10 9 8 7 6 5 4 3 2 1

Illustrations by Nicole Kaufman

While the publisher believes the information used in creating this book to be reliable, the medical
field changes rapidly and there are new developments almost daily. The publisher cannot guarantee
the accuracy, adequacy, or the completeness of the information contained in this book and must
disclaim all warranties, expressed or implied, regarding the information. The publisher also cannot
assume any responsibility for use of this book, and any use by a reader is at the reader's own risk.
This book is not intended to be a substitute for professional medical advice, and any user of this book
should always check with a licensed physician before adopting any particular course of treatment.

For information about custom editions, special sales, premium and corporate purchases, please
contact the Sterling Special Sales Department at 800-805-5489 or specialsales@sterlingpub.com.

Contents

PART THREE

Baby Steps

PART FOUR

Baby Is Born

PART FIVE
PERSONAL DIRECTORY

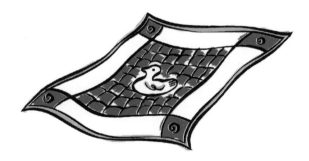

Introduction

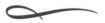

*C*ongratulations, and welcome to the magical world of pregnancy! It's hard to believe that in 266 days, give or take a few, what began as a pair of cells inside you will become an entire person. The coming months will bring a great amount of change—not only to your body, but to your lifestyle and schedule as well. There's much to do, and keeping track of all the information and plans can seem overwhelming at times.

The *Great Expectations Pregnancy Journal & Planner* has been designed to help make all of the details more manageable. Here, you can note any physical sensations you're experiencing, keep track of your diet and fitness activity, write down any questions you want to ask your care provider, and record any results and instructions you receive at your medical appointments. This way, you can stay organized and keep all of your pregnancy-related information in one place. There are also to-do lists; suggested questions to ask when looking for care providers, checking out childcare options, and touring a birthing facility; factors to consider when devising a birth plan; and a host of other tools to help you prepare for baby's arrival. And once your baby has arrived, you'll have this wonderful document to help you remember your pregnancy journey—and to guide you if you become pregnant again someday.

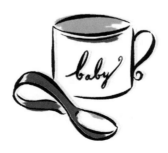

Timeline of Things to Do

The following brief summary of things to do during pregnancy is a general guideline to help you plan ahead.

First Trimester

☐ Begin reading pregnancy books and magazines and visiting reputable Web sites to become well informed about the process you'll be going through; at the same time, avoid "reality" birth shows and medical dramas like last week's fish, because they make hours of hard work look like it takes minutes, and they focus on high-tension drama rather than presenting birth as a healthy experience

☐ Interview several obstetricians, midwives, or family practitioners to find the one best suited to your physical and emotional needs (questions to ask can be found on page 96)

☐ Inform your healthcare provider of any medications, vitamins, or herbal supplements that you are currently taking or that you took before you found out you were pregnant

☐ Start taking the prenatal vitamins recommended by your care provider

☐ Clean out your medicine cabinets; remove old or unsafe medications

☐ Clean out your refrigerator, freezer, and pantry; remove old or unappealing food

☐ Assess your workplace for hazards or toxins

☐ Enroll in a prenatal exercise class and/or create a plan to get at least 30 minutes of exercise daily (ask your healthcare provider about exercise precautions first)

☐ Start Kegel exercises to strengthen your pelvic floor

☐ Make sure that your care provider has your most up-to-date medical records, including all pertaining to any past births or surgeries

Second Trimester

☐ Tell your friends, employer, children, and coworkers that you're pregnant, if you haven't already

☐ Keep up your Kegels and your daily 30-minute exercise routine, as approved by your healthcare provider

☐ Investigate pediatricians or physicians in family practice for your baby, and set up initial consultations to choose the one who's the best fit for you and your child (see page 136 for some questions you might want to ask)

☐ Research and schedule childbirth classes (see page 144 for some questions you may want to ask)

☐ Select the hospital or birth center where you wish to give birth by taking tours of the facilities, if your care provider delivers at more than one place

☐ Start exploring your childcare options, if you plan to return to work after your baby arrives (questions to ask begin on page 176)

☐ Shop for maternity wear (see the checklist of suggested items on page 160)

☐ Begin thinking of "boy" and "girl" names (see the back of the tabbed divider in Part Four for some tips)

☐ Start preparing any other children you have for the changes your body will be going through and for having a new baby in the house

☐ Inform your insurance company that you're pregnant and ask how to add your baby to your policy (you can contact the company by calling the customer service number on your insurance card)

☐ Sign up for baby clubs on baby product–sponsored Web sites, if you want direct-mail coupons and freebies

☐ Consider attending monthly La Leche League meetings to get practical breastfeeding information and support, if you plan to breastfeed (groups are often listed in the white pages of the telephone directory, or you can locate leaders online at www.LaLecheLeague.org)

☐ Complete home-remodeling jobs by the end of this trimester (especially strong-smelling projects like painting and carpeting your baby's sleeping area and other areas of the home) to give the spaces a chance to air out completely before the baby arrives; be sure to wear an industrial-quality face mask and keep work areas well ventilated, particularly when using products that contain volatile compounds, such as petroleum-based paint thinners and sprays; avoid perching on ladders, as your changing center of gravity can make you more prone to falls

☐ If your home was built before 1978, have flaking or chipped indoor paint professionally removed to minimize your inhalation or ingestion of toxic lead dust and chips

☐ Schedule plenty of quality time with your partner and other family members

Third Trimester

☐ Tour the hospital/birth center you plan to use, if you haven't done so already

☐ Ask for preadmission forms from the healthcare facility where you'll be delivering if you haven't already, and fill them out in advance so that you won't have to do it when you're in labor

☐ Finalize your maternity-leave arrangements with your employer, if you work and plan to return to your job

☐ Meet with a financial planner to discuss long-term goals, such as saving for your child's education; you may also want to talk with an insurance agent about obtaining a life insurance policy or increasing your current coverage

☐ Contact an attorney about getting your will in order

☐ Consider hiring a labor assistant (doula) to help you through birth, as well as a postpartum doula to assist you in the weeks that follow

☐ Study baby products, and create a master list of the specific items you want, noting model names and numbers (see page 161 for a list of basic necessities, as well as other gear and clothing you may want to consider)

☐ Register for baby items at stores after doing your research

☐ Buy stationery or cards to write thank-you notes for baby gifts (and use them)

☐ Save receipts for baby items, including ones you receive as gifts, and put all these slips in one easy-to-remember place

☐ Browse consignment shops that buy and sell gently used baby clothes and gear; but purchase your baby's crib mattress and car seat new for maximum safety

☐ Acquire any essentials that you didn't get as gifts

☐ Safely install your baby's car seat facing rearward in the backseat of your car by following both the directions that come with the seat and those printed in your auto owner's manual; have the installation inspected at your local police or fire department to make sure it's correct

☐ Create a designated mail area where you can organize bills, stamps, and correspondence

☐ Organize all of your important documents, such as vehicle records, bank statements, insurance information, birth certificates, and passports, in an easy-to-find spot so that your partner will be able to locate them if they're needed while you're busy with the baby

☐ Line up extra household help for baby's first month

☐ Collect menus from nearby restaurants offering takeout or delivery, and circle your favorite dishes

☐ Stock up on household supplies as well as frozen and canned foods and other nonperishables (see the list on page 194 for suggestions)

☐ Create a written birth plan, and discuss your wishes with your care provider (see page 154 for issues to consider)

☐ Kegel, Kegel, Kegel!

☐ Determine who will drive you to the healthcare facility when you go into labor (and appoint a backup driver just in case)

☐ Do a practice drive to the hospital/birth center; time the trip, and write down the directions to keep in your purse (you'll find space for recording this information on page 223)

☐ Arrange for someone to care for your other children and/or your pets and to tend to plants, newspapers, and mail while you're off having the baby

☐ Pack your bag with the things you want to bring to the healthcare facility when it's time to have the baby (see page 174)

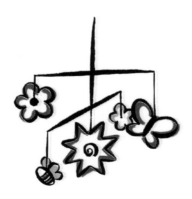

PART ONE

Week-by-
Week
Tracker

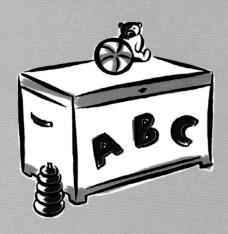

Milestones in Baby Development

The section below highlights some of the milestones of a baby's development in utero. The weeks used here indicate gestational age, which is calculated according to the first day of your last period (for a more in-depth explanation of this, see page 13). Note that the time frames given for the events mentioned here are general estimates, as individual rates of development vary somewhat from baby to baby, especially in the later weeks.

First Trimester
Week 4: Between days 21 and 24 after conception, a tube that will become the heart will start circulating the embryo's own blood.

Week 5: The beginnings of the eyes, ears, tongue, lungs, and spinal cord appear this week. What will become the arms manifest themselves as tiny buds.

Week 6: The legs appear as buds, just as the arms did in the previous week.

Week 8: All of the essential organs have begun to form by this point.

Week 9: The embryo is now known as a fetus. Brain waves can be detected.

Week 10: Fetal heartbeat can usually be detected by a handheld Doppler.

Week 11: The fetus can turn over, hiccup, stretch, and flex her fingers.

Second Trimester
Week 14: Teeth begin to form under the gum line, and hair starts to grow on the head. Hearing has developed to the point where the fetus can be startled by loud sounds.

Week 17: Genitalia can be seen via ultrasound.

Week 18: With lots of amniotic fluid to play in, and good muscle control, the baby is very active; she can suck her thumb, cross and uncross her legs, even do somersaults.

Week 24: The baby may kick in response to sounds outside the womb.

Third Trimester
Week 28: The baby's eyes, which were previously covered by sealed eyelids, can now open and close.

Week 31: With every passing week, the baby's nervous system is better able to control her bodily functions, such as breathing and temperature regulation.

Week 38: The baby is fully developed, though still gaining weight and adding connections between neurons in the brain, an activity that continues after birth.

Make a Note of It

Welcome to your personal week-by-week pregnancy tracker. Keeping track of how far along you are in your pregnancy can be confusing, because medical professionals start counting from the first day of your last menstrual period (LMP). In reality, you probably didn't conceive until about two weeks after that.

This section gives you two sets of ages. The main heading is the gestational age, which counts from the first day of your last period and will be the number your doctor will use. Also included is the fetal age, which is an approximation of how long it's been since the day of conception. While pregnancy lasts 40 weeks according to the gestational calendar, there are actually about 38 weeks (or about 266 days) from conception to birth.

To get started, grab a pen and write your due date on the first day of Week 40 in the tracker section (see page 88). Then work backward, adding dates to the header of each week until you get to the beginning of the section (for your convenience, we've included dated reference calendars on page 15). The tracker begins with Week 4, because that's the week of your first missed period and usually the earliest that most women will have high enough levels of pregnancy hormone to be detected by most pregnancy tests.

Note that babies tend not to arrive on the day they're due. Your baby could make his entrance into the world two weeks before or after the estimated due date and still be considered "on time." Still, planning your pregnancy around the estimated delivery date will give you a general window for accomplishing things in preparation for your baby.

This section allows you to track a variety of aspects of your pregnancy, from the emotional to the physical. Plus, to help you stay organized, there is space for you to jot down weekly to-do lists. Also provided are general length and weight estimates to give you an idea of a baby's size each week. During the first weeks of your pregnancy, the embryo destined to turn into your baby will be so miniscule that it could practically fit on the head of a pin. Familiar weight measurements such as ounces and pounds simply aren't precise enough to describe something so small. By about Week 8, though, the embryo will become heavy enough to be measured in grams. Around Week 11 the approximate weight can easily be expressed in terms of ounces, and by about Week 23, the approximate weight finally reaches the one-pound mark. Like weights, length measurements for fetuses are simply averages. Starting around Week 9, the length will generally be expressed as being "from crown to rump." That's because the baby's legs are curled into the body. At Week 20, as the baby begins to stretch out, measurements are from crown to heel. Again, these measurements are just averages, as individual growth rates and sizes vary. By delivery, your baby could weigh as little as five pounds or more than nine pounds and still be considered normal. So don't be concerned if your care provider tells you that your baby is somewhat smaller or larger than the tracker indicates.

Also included is space for you to record notes about any exercise that you're doing. Exercise has numerous benefits for most pregnant women; however, do ask your care provider beforehand if there are any activities you should avoid or specific instructions you should follow. This section also includes a place for nutrition notes if you want to keep track of your meals or reactions to foods.

From Week 20 on, there's space for you to make notes on your baby's activity, should you wish to do so. If you've been pregnant before or you're particularly sensitive, you may feel movement sooner, as early as Week 16, as the result of your baby's largest bones becoming harder. If you're overweight, it may take you a little longer. Babies are typically most active at night and after you've eaten. Don't worry about counting how many kicks per hour you feel (unless your care provider tells you to). What's important is that you feel the baby move at least once a day, that you get used to and keep track of how much your baby moves each day, and that the level of activity doesn't decrease, especially in the third trimester. If you don't feel the baby move like he normally does, tell your care provider. Bear in mind that at the very end of the pregnancy, the baby may move a bit less because of how crowded it's getting inside the uterus. Still, if the baby is moving less than usual, make sure to tell your care provider.

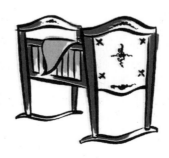

2005

JANUARY
```
S  M  T  W  T  F  S
               1
2  3  4  5  6  7  8
9  10 11 12 13 14 15
16 17 18 19 20 21 22
23 24 25 26 27 28 29
30 31
```

FEBRUARY
```
S  M  T  W  T  F  S
      1  2  3  4  5
6  7  8  9  10 11 12
13 14 15 16 17 18 19
20 21 22 23 24 25 26
27 28
```

MARCH
```
S  M  T  W  T  F  S
      1  2  3  4  5
6  7  8  9  10 11 12
13 14 15 16 17 18 19
20 21 22 23 24 25 26
27 28 29 30 31
```

APRIL
```
S  M  T  W  T  F  S
                  1  2
3  4  5  6  7  8  9
10 11 12 13 14 15 16
17 18 19 20 21 22 23
24 25 26 27 28 29 30
```

MAY
```
S  M  T  W  T  F  S
1  2  3  4  5  6  7
8  9  10 11 12 13 14
15 16 17 18 19 20 21
22 23 24 25 26 27 28
29 30 31
```

JUNE
```
S  M  T  W  T  F  S
         1  2  3  4
5  6  7  8  9  10 11
12 13 14 15 16 17 18
19 20 21 22 23 24 25
26 27 28 29 30
```

JULY
```
S  M  T  W  T  F  S
                  1  2
3  4  5  6  7  8  9
10 11 12 13 14 15 16
17 18 19 20 21 22 23
24 25 26 27 28 29 30
31
```

AUGUST
```
S  M  T  W  T  F  S
   1  2  3  4  5  6
7  8  9  10 11 12 13
14 15 16 17 18 19 20
21 22 23 24 25 26 27
28 29 30 31
```

SEPTEMBER
```
S  M  T  W  T  F  S
            1  2  3
4  5  6  7  8  9  10
11 12 13 14 15 16 17
18 19 20 21 22 23 24
25 26 27 28 29 30
```

OCTOBER
```
S  M  T  W  T  F  S
                  1
2  3  4  5  6  7  8
9  10 11 12 13 14 15
16 17 18 19 20 21 22
23 24 25 26 27 28 29
30 31
```

NOVEMBER
```
S  M  T  W  T  F  S
      1  2  3  4  5
6  7  8  9  10 11 12
13 14 15 16 17 18 19
20 21 22 23 24 25 26
27 28 29 30
```

DECEMBER
```
S  M  T  W  T  F  S
            1  2  3
4  5  6  7  8  9  10
11 12 13 14 15 16 17
18 19 20 21 22 23 24
25 26 27 28 29 30 31
```

2006

JANUARY
```
S  M  T  W  T  F  S
1  2  3  4  5  6  7
8  9  10 11 12 13 14
15 16 17 18 19 20 21
22 23 24 25 26 27 28
29 30 31
```

FEBRUARY
```
S  M  T  W  T  F  S
         1  2  3  4
5  6  7  8  9  10 11
12 13 14 15 16 17 18
19 20 21 22 23 24 25
26 27 28
```

MARCH
```
S  M  T  W  T  F  S
         1  2  3  4
5  6  7  8  9  10 11
12 13 14 15 16 17 18
19 20 21 22 23 24 25
26 27 28 29 30 31
```

APRIL
```
S  M  T  W  T  F  S
                  1
2  3  4  5  6  7  8
9  10 11 12 13 14 15
16 17 18 19 20 21 22
23 24 25 26 27 28 29
30
```

MAY
```
S  M  T  W  T  F  S
   1  2  3  4  5  6
7  8  9  10 11 12 13
14 15 16 17 18 19 20
21 22 23 24 25 26 27
28 29 30 31
```

JUNE
```
S  M  T  W  T  F  S
            1  2  3
4  5  6  7  8  9  10
11 12 13 14 15 16 17
18 19 20 21 22 23 24
25 26 27 28 29 30
```

JULY
```
S  M  T  W  T  F  S
                  1
2  3  4  5  6  7  8
9  10 11 12 13 14 15
16 17 18 19 20 21 22
23 24 25 26 27 28 29
30 31
```

AUGUST
```
S  M  T  W  T  F  S
      1  2  3  4  5
6  7  8  9  10 11 12
13 14 15 16 17 18 19
20 21 22 23 24 25 26
27 28 29 30 31
```

SEPTEMBER
```
S  M  T  W  T  F  S
               1  2
3  4  5  6  7  8  9
10 11 12 13 14 15 16
17 18 19 20 21 22 23
24 25 26 27 28 29 30
```

OCTOBER
```
S  M  T  W  T  F  S
1  2  3  4  5  6  7
8  9  10 11 12 13 14
15 16 17 18 19 20 21
22 23 24 25 26 27 28
29 30 31
```

NOVEMBER
```
S  M  T  W  T  F  S
         1  2  3  4
5  6  7  8  9  10 11
12 13 14 15 16 17 18
19 20 21 22 23 24 25
26 27 28 29 30
```

DECEMBER
```
S  M  T  W  T  F  S
                  1  2
3  4  5  6  7  8  9
10 11 12 13 14 15 16
17 18 19 20 21 22 23
24 25 26 27 28 29 30
31
```

2007

JANUARY
```
S  M  T  W  T  F  S
   1  2  3  4  5  6
7  8  9  10 11 12 13
14 15 16 17 18 19 20
21 22 23 24 25 26 27
28 29 30 31
```

FEBRUARY
```
S  M  T  W  T  F  S
            1  2  3
4  5  6  7  8  9  10
11 12 13 14 15 16 17
18 19 20 21 22 23 24
25 26 27 28
```

MARCH
```
S  M  T  W  T  F  S
            1  2  3
4  5  6  7  8  9  10
11 12 13 14 15 16 17
18 19 20 21 22 23 24
25 26 27 28 29 30 31
```

APRIL
```
S  M  T  W  T  F  S
1  2  3  4  5  6  7
8  9  10 11 12 13 14
15 16 17 18 19 20 21
22 23 24 25 26 27 28
29 30
```

MAY
```
S  M  T  W  T  F  S
      1  2  3  4  5
6  7  8  9  10 11 12
13 14 15 16 17 18 19
20 21 22 23 24 25 26
27 28 29 30 31
```

JUNE
```
S  M  T  W  T  F  S
                  1  2
3  4  5  6  7  8  9
10 11 12 13 14 15 16
17 18 19 20 21 22 23
24 25 26 27 28 29 30
```

JULY
```
S  M  T  W  T  F  S
1  2  3  4  5  6  7
8  9  10 11 12 13 14
15 16 17 18 19 20 21
22 23 24 25 26 27 28
29 30 31
```

AUGUST
```
S  M  T  W  T  F  S
         1  2  3  4
5  6  7  8  9  10 11
12 13 14 15 16 17 18
19 20 21 22 23 24 25
26 27 28 29 30 31
```

SEPTEMBER
```
S  M  T  W  T  F  S
                  1
2  3  4  5  6  7  8
9  10 11 12 13 14 15
16 17 18 19 20 21 22
23 24 25 26 27 28 29
30
```

OCTOBER
```
S  M  T  W  T  F  S
   1  2  3  4  5  6
7  8  9  10 11 12 13
14 15 16 17 18 19 20
21 22 23 24 25 26 27
28 29 30 31
```

NOVEMBER
```
S  M  T  W  T  F  S
            1  2  3
4  5  6  7  8  9  10
11 12 13 14 15 16 17
18 19 20 21 22 23 24
25 26 27 28 29 30
```

DECEMBER
```
S  M  T  W  T  F  S
                  1
2  3  4  5  6  7  8
9  10 11 12 13 14 15
16 17 18 19 20 21 22
23 24 25 26 27 28 29
30 31
```

Week 4

Dates: _____ **to** _____

Countdown: *36 to 35 weeks (251 to 245 days) until your due date*
Fetal age: *15 to 21 days*
Size of embryo: *Barely visible to the naked eye*

My mood:

How my body feels:

Exercise/activities:

First Trimester

Dreams:

Nutrition notes:

Things to do this week:

Week 5

Dates: _____ **to** _____

Countdown: *35 to 34 weeks (244 to 238 days) until your due date*
Fetal age: *22 to 28 days*
Length: *About 2 millimeters*

My mood:

How my body feels:

Exercise/activities:

First Trimester

Dreams:

Nutrition notes:

Things to do this week:

Week 6

Dates: _____ **to** _____

Countdown: *34 to 33 weeks (237 to 231 days) until your due date*
Fetal age: *29 to 35 days*
Length: *About 5 to 7 millimeters*

My mood:

How my body feels:

Exercise/activities:

First Trimester

Dreams:

Nutrition notes:

Things to do this week:

Week 7

Dates: _____ **to** _____

Countdown: *33 to 32 weeks (230 to 224 days) until your due date*
Fetal age: *36 to 42 days*
Length: *About 13 millimeters*

My mood:

How my body feels:

Exercise/activities:

First Trimester

Dreams:

Nutrition notes:

Things to do this week:

Week 8   **Dates:** _____ **to** _____

Countdown: *32 to 31 weeks (223 to 217 days) until your due date*
Fetal age: *43 to 49 days*
Length: *1/2 to 3/4 inch*   **Weight:** *About 1 gram*

My mood:

How my body feels:

Exercise/activities:

First Trimester

Dreams:

Nutrition notes:

Things to do this week:

Week 9   Dates: _____ to _____

Countdown: *31 to 30 weeks (216 to 210 days) until your due date*
Fetal age: *50 to 56 days*
Length: *About ¾ inch from crown to rump*   **Weight:** *About 2 grams*

My mood:

How my body feels:

Exercise/activities:

First Trimester

Dreams:

Nutrition notes:

Things to do this week:

Week 10   Dates: _____ to _____

Countdown: *30 to 29 weeks (209 to 203 days) until your due date*
Fetal age: *57 to 63 days*
Length: *About 1 inch from crown to rump*   **Weight:** *About 5 grams*

My mood:

How my body feels:

Exercise/activities:

First Trimester

Dreams:

Nutrition notes:

Things to do this week:

Week 11

Dates: _____ **to** _____

Countdown: *29 to 28 weeks (202 to 196 days) until your due date*
Fetal age: *64 to 70 days*
Length: *About 1³/₄ inches from crown to rump*   **Weight:** *About ¹/₃ ounce*

My mood:

How my body feels:

Exercise/activities:

First Trimester

Dreams:

Nutrition notes:

Things to do this week:

Week 12   Dates: _____ to _____

Countdown: *28 to 27 weeks (195 to 189 days) until your due date*
Fetal age: *71 to 77 days*
Length: *About 2½ inches from crown to rump*   **Weight:** *About ½ ounce*

My mood:

How my body feels:

Exercise/activities:

First Trimester

Dreams:

Nutrition notes:

Things to do this week:

Week 13

Dates: _____ **to** _____

Countdown: *27 to 26 weeks (188 to 182 days) until your due date*
Fetal age: *78 to 84 days*
Length: *About 3 inches from crown to rump*   **Weight:** *About 1 ounce*

My mood:

How my body feels:

Exercise/activities:

First Trimester

Dreams:

Nutrition notes:

Things to do this week:

Week 14

Dates: _____ **to** _____

Countdown: *26 to 25 weeks (181 to 175 days) until your due date*
Fetal age: *85 to 91 days*
Length: *About 3¹/₂ inches from crown to rump*   **Weight:** *About 1¹/₂ ounces*

My mood:

How my body feels:

Exercise/activities:

Second Trimester

Dreams:

Nutrition notes:

Things to do this week:

Week 15

Dates: _____ **to** _____

Countdown: *25 to 24 weeks (174 to 168 days) until your due date*
Fetal age: *92 to 98 days*
Length: *About 4 inches from crown to rump*   **Weight:** *About 2 ounces*

My mood:

How my body feels:

Exercise/activities:

Second Trimester

Dreams:

Nutrition notes:

Things to do this week:

Week 16

Dates: _____ to _____

Countdown: *24 to 23 weeks (167 to 161 days) until your due date*
Fetal age: *99 to 105 days*
Length: *About 4½ inches from crown to rump*   **Weight:** *About 2.8 ounces*

My mood:

How my body feels:

Exercise/activities:

Second Trimester

Dreams:

Nutrition notes:

Things to do this week:

Week 17

Dates: _____ **to** _____

Countdown: *23 to 22 weeks (160 to 154 days) until your due date*
Fetal age: *106 to 112 days*
Length: *About 5 inches from crown to rump*   **Weight:** *About 4 ounces*

My mood:

How my body feels:

Exercise/activities:

Second Trimester

Dreams:

Nutrition notes:

Things to do this week:

Week 18   Dates: _____ to _____

Countdown: *22 to 21 weeks (153 to 147 days) until your due date*
Fetal age: *113 to 119 days*
Length: *About 5 1/2 inches from crown to rump*
Weight: *A little more than 5 ounces*

My mood:

How my body feels:

Exercise/activities:

Second Trimester

Dreams:

Nutrition notes:

Things to do this week:

Week 19

Dates: _____ **to** _____

Countdown: *21 to 20 weeks (146 to 140 days) until your due date*
Fetal age: *120 to 126 days*
Length: *About 6 inches from crown to rump*   **Weight:** *About 7 ounces*

My mood:

How my body feels:

Exercise/activities:

Second Trimester

Dreams:

Nutrition notes:

Things to do this week:

Week 20   Dates: _____ to _____

Countdown: *20 to 19 weeks (139 to 133 days) until your due date*
Fetal age: *127 to 133 days*
Length: *About 6½ inches from crown to rump; about 10 inches from crown to heel*   **Weight:** *About 9 ounces*

My mood:

How my body feels:

Exercise/activities:

Second Trimester

Dreams:

Nutrition notes:

Things to do this week:

Baby's activity:

Week 21   Dates: _____ to _____

Countdown: *19 to 18 weeks (132 to 126 days) until your due date*
Fetal age: *134 to 140 days*
Length: *About 7 inches from crown to rump; about 10½ inches from crown to heel*   **Weight:** *About 10½ ounces*

My mood:

How my body feels:

Exercise/activities:

Second Trimester

Dreams:

Nutrition notes:

Things to do this week:

Baby's activity:

Week 22

Dates: _____ **to** _____

Countdown: *18 to 17 weeks (125 to 119 days) until your due date*
Fetal age: *141 to 147 days*
Length: *About 11 inches from crown to heel*   **Weight:** *About 15 ounces*

My mood:

How my body feels:

Exercise/activities:

Second Trimester

Dreams:

Nutrition notes:

Things to do this week:

Baby's activity:

Week 23

Dates: _____ **to** _____

Countdown: *17 to 16 weeks (118 to 112 days) until your due date*
Fetal age: *148 to 154 days*
Length: *About 11½ inches from crown to heel*   **Weight:** *About 1 pound*

My mood:

How my body feels:

Exercise/activities:

Second Trimester

Dreams:

Nutrition notes:

Things to do this week:

Baby's activity:

Week 24   Dates: _____ to _____

Countdown: *16 to 15 weeks (111 to 105 days) until your due date*
Fetal age: *155 to 161 days*
Length: *About 12 inches from crown to heel*   **Weight:** *About 1 1/4 pounds*

My mood:

How my body feels:

Exercise/activities:

Second Trimester

Dreams:

Nutrition notes:

Things to do this week:

Baby's activity:

Week 25   Dates: _____ to _____

Countdown: *15 to 14 weeks (104 to 98 days) until your due date*
Fetal age: *162 to 168 days*
Length: *About 13³/₄ inches from crown to heel*   **Weight:** *1¹/₃ pounds*

My mood:

How my body feels:

Exercise/activities:

Third Trimester

Dreams:

Nutrition notes:

Things to do this week:

Baby's activity:

Week 26   Dates: _____ to _____

Countdown: *14 to 13 weeks (97 to 91 days) until your due date*
Fetal age: *169 to 175 days*
Length: *About 14 inches from crown to heel*   **Weight:** *About 1½ pounds*

My mood:

How my body feels:

Exercise/activities:

Third Trimester

Dreams:

Nutrition notes:

Things to do this week:

Baby's activity:

Week 27   Dates: _____ to _____

Countdown: *13 to 12 weeks (90 to 84 days) until your due date*
Fetal age: *176 to 182 days*
Length: *About 14½ inches from crown to heel*   **Weight:** *About 2 pounds*

My mood:

How my body feels:

Exercise/activities:

Third Trimester

Dreams:

Nutrition notes:

Things to do this week:

Baby's activity:

Week 28

Dates: _____ **to** _____

Countdown: *12 to 11 weeks (83 to 77 days) until your due date*
Fetal age: *183 to 189 days*
Length: *About 15 inches from crown to heel*   **Weight:** *About 2½ pounds*

My mood:

How my body feels:

Exercise/activities:

Third Trimester

Dreams:

Nutrition notes:

Things to do this week:

Baby's activity:

Week 29   Dates: _____ to _____

Countdown: *11 to 10 weeks (76 to 70 days) until your due date*
Fetal age: *190 to 196 days*
Length: *About 15½ inches from crown to heel*   **Weight:** *About 2¾ pounds*

My mood:

How my body feels:

Exercise/activities:

Third Trimester

Dreams:

Nutrition notes:

Things to do this week:

Baby's activity:

Week 30   Dates: _____ to _____

Countdown: *10 to 9 weeks (69 to 63 days) until your due date*
Fetal age: *197 to 203 days*
Length: *About 15¾ inches from crown to heel*   **Weight:** *About 3 pounds*

My mood:

How my body feels:

Exercise/activities:

Third Trimester

Dreams:

Nutrition notes:

Things to do this week:

Baby's activity:

Week 31

Dates: _____ **to** _____

Countdown: *9 to 8 weeks (62 to 56 days) until your due date*
Fetal age: *204 to 210 days*
Length: *About 16 inches from crown to heel*   **Weight:** *About 3 1/3 pounds*

My mood:

How my body feels:

Exercise/activities:

Third Trimester

Dreams:

Nutrition notes:

Things to do this week:

Baby's activity:

Week 32   Dates: _____ to _____

Countdown: *8 to 7 weeks (55 to 49 days) until your due date*
Fetal age: *211 to 217 days*
Length: *About 16½ inches from crown to heel*   **Weight:** *About 4 pounds*

My mood:

How my body feels:

Exercise/activities:

Third Trimester

Dreams:

Nutrition notes:

Things to do this week:

Baby's activity:

Week 33   Dates: _____ to _____

Countdown: *7 to 6 weeks (48 to 42 days) until your due date*
Fetal age: *218 to 224 days*
Length: *About 17¼ inches from crown to heel*   **Weight:** *About 4½ pounds*

My mood:

How my body feels:

Exercise/activities:

Third Trimester

Dreams:

Nutrition notes:

Things to do this week:

Baby's activity:

Week 34

Dates: _____ **to** _____

Countdown: *6 to 5 weeks (41 to 35 days) until your due date*
Fetal age: *225 to 231 days*
Length: *About 17³/4 inches from crown to heel*   **Weight:** *About 5 pounds*

My mood:

How my body feels:

Exercise/activities:

Third Trimester

Dreams:

Nutrition notes:

Things to do this week:

Baby's activity:

Week 35

Dates: _____ **to** _____

Countdown: *5 to 4 weeks (34 to 28 days) until your due date*
Fetal age: *232 to 238 days*
Length: *About 18 inches from crown to heel* **Weight:** *About 5 1/4 pounds*

My mood:

How my body feels:

Exercise/activities:

Third Trimester

Dreams:

Nutrition notes:

Things to do this week:

Baby's activity:

Week 36   Dates: _____ to _____

Countdown: *4 to 3 weeks (27 to 21 days) until your due date*
Fetal age: *239 to 245 days*
Length: *About 18³/₄ inches from crown to heel*   **Weight:** *About 6 pounds*

My mood:

How my body feels:

Exercise/activities:

Third Trimester

Dreams:

Nutrition notes:

Things to do this week:

Baby's activity:

Week 37

Dates: _____ **to** _____

Countdown: *3 to 2 weeks (20 to 14 days) until your due date*
Fetal age: *246 to 252 days*
Length: *About 19 inches from crown to heel*   **Weight:** *About 6½ pounds*

My mood:

How my body feels:

Exercise/activities:

Third Trimester

Dreams:

Nutrition notes:

Things to do this week:

Baby's activity:

Week 38

Dates: _____ **to** _____

Countdown: *2 weeks to 1 week (13 to 7 days) until your due date*
Fetal age: *253 to 259 days*
Length: *19½ inches on average from crown to heel, though between 17 and 23 inches is normal* **Weight:** *About 6¾ pounds*

My mood:

How my body feels:

Exercise/activities:

Third Trimester

Dreams:

Nutrition notes:

Things to do this week:

Baby's activity:

Week 39

Dates: _____ **to** _____

Countdown: *7 to 0 days until your due date*
Fetal age: *260 to 266 days*
Length: *About 20 inches from crown to heel*
Weight: *Average birth weight is 7 1/2 pounds*

My mood:

How my body feels:

Exercise/activities:

Third Trimester

Dreams:

Nutrition notes:

Things to do this week:

Baby's activity:

Week 40

Dates: _____ **to** _____

Countdown: *0 to 7 days after your due date*
Fetal age: *267 to 273 days*
Length: *About 20 inches from crown to heel*   **Weight:** *Around 7³/4 pounds*
Generally, a baby gains about an extra 1/4 to 1/2 pound for every week past the due date, though she will probably not get much taller.

My mood:

How my body feels:

Exercise/activities:

Third Trimester

Dreams:

Nutrition notes:

Things to do this week:

Baby's activity:

Week 41

Dates: _____ **to** _____

Countdown: *8 to 14 days after your due date*
Fetal age: *274 to 280 days*
Length: *About 20 inches from crown to heel* **Weight:** *Around 8 pounds*

My mood:

How my body feels:

Exercise/activities:

Third Trimester

Dreams:

Nutrition notes:

Things to do this week:

Baby's activity:

PART TWO

Medical
Record
Keeper

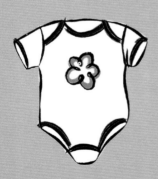

Choosing Your Care Provider

Only one person is going to deliver your baby—you! But the right care provider can make a big difference in how comfortable and safe your birth is. You're bestowing a lot of trust on this person, and you'll be spending a lot of time with her over the next year. Take time to shop around until you find a family practitioner, obstetrician, or midwife who is skilled, has good judgment, and makes you feel at ease.

A good care provider:

❖ answers your questions thoroughly and with respect, regardless of how small or big the issue
❖ doesn't make you feel rushed during appointments
❖ doesn't make you wait for your appointment for longer than 30 minutes (unless she's attending to an emergency)
❖ advises you without being judgmental
❖ explains what she is doing and why
❖ warns you beforehand if a procedure is going to be unpleasant
❖ explains the risks and benefits of any test or procedure clearly
❖ is familiar with health concerns particular to your ethnicity and medical history
❖ refers you to a specialist if you have a condition beyond her particular expertise
❖ respects your personal and/or religious beliefs
❖ belongs to a practice where you feel comfortable with the other doctors or midwives (if she's not alone in her practice)
❖ delivers at a hospital or birth center that is convenient to your home and that offers the pain relief options, amenities, and facilities you prefer
❖ makes you feel comfortable

A good care provider's office staff:

❖ makes sure your calls are returned promptly
❖ does their best to let you know beforehand what your insurance company will and won't pay for
❖ makes sure a copy of your medical records is on file at your hospital or birth center before you deliver

Managing Your Medical Care

This chapter is devoted to your medical care. Here, you'll find prepared interviews to help you in your selection of healthcare providers, pages to record personal medical information, and a list of considerations for formulating a birth plan.

Starting on page 115, there are sheets for making notes regarding your prenatal appointments. You can use these not only to record information you receive during your exams, but also to write down ahead of time any questions you want to ask your care provider during your visit. If you need more of these appointment sheets, simply make photocopies and keep them in the pocket provided at the end of this book. In addition, there are pages for noting information about your medical tests, as well as a place to record the details from your postpartum exam, which usually occurs about six weeks after giving birth.

One of the first things you'll need to do is find a healthcare provider to monitor your pregnancy and deliver your baby (see page 96). You'll also need to find a pediatrician for your bundle of joy. The best time to select a pediatrician is between the third and seventh months of your pregnancy, with earlier being better if your pregnancy is high-risk. Friends, family, your childbirth educator, your insurance company, and your own physician can help you locate pediatricians in your area. For a list of questions you might want to ask when trying to choose a doctor for your baby, turn to page 136. When you go to meet with a prospective pediatrician, pay attention not only to your comfort level with the doctor but also to the way the receptionist and the rest of the staff act toward you and other parents. Once your child is under the care of a pediatrician, you may spend as much time interacting with the staff as you do with the doctor. Consider, too, how you feel about the pediatrician as a care provider for your child over the long term—not just while he's a baby.

You may also want to look into childbirth classes, which can be a great experience, even if you've had a baby before. Most hospitals and birth centers offer these. You can also locate a class by contacting one of the following major organizations: the International Childbirth Education Association (www.icea.org), the American Academy of Husband-Coached Childbirth® (the Bradley Method®, www.bradleybirth.com), or Lamaze® International (www.lamaze.org). All three groups are committed to parental participation in the birth process and reducing the need for interventions. Once you locate a class, contact the instructor about the details (see the list of questions on page 144). An added bonus of attending childbirth classes is that it gives you the opportunity to talk to other expectant parents and meet people whose babies will be the same age as yours (so that you can keep in touch with these people, we've provided space in the directory at the end of this book for you to fill in their contact information [see page 222]).

Last but not least, having a professional labor-support person in the delivery room is a great idea, especially if you're giving birth in a hospital where labor and delivery nurses may change shifts. The services of such a person can both assist you and take pressure off your family and friends. Note that many hospitals will supply a labor assistant if you request one. You can also find the names and contact information for doulas on www.dona.org, on www.icea.org, and on other national doula listings on the Internet. If you opt to hire your own, see page 148 for some questions you may want to ask.

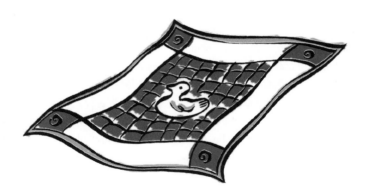

Thoughts/Information

Questions to Ask an Obstetrician/Midwife/Family Practitioner

Following are some questions you may want to ask when deciding on a healthcare provider for your pregnancy.

	Candidate I
Name/practice:	
Address:	
Phone:	
Fax:	
❖ Does your practice accept my health insurance?	
❖ What are your daily office hours?	
❖ What are your hours on weekends and holidays, if any?	
❖ As far as you know, will you be in town in the two weeks before and the two weeks after my due date?	
❖ Can I call your office when I have questions? Are there certain hours when it's best to call if I have questions that aren't urgent?	
❖ How soon can I expect to have my calls returned?	
❖ What hospital(s) or birth center(s) are you affiliated with?	
❖ Do I have a choice regarding where I give birth?	
❖ How long have you been in practice?	

Candidate II	Candidate III

	Candidate I
❖ About how many babies do you deliver a month? *Fewer than 30 is best.*	
❖ How many babies have you delivered over the course of your career? Have you lost any?	
❖ Tell me about your degrees and special training.	
❖ What is your general philosophy regarding pregnancy and birth?	
❖ What would cause you to classify my pregnancy as "high-risk"?	
❖ At what point would you recommend the services of a specialist in maternal-fetal medicine?	
❖ How many other family practitioners, obstetricians, and/or midwives are in the practice? Will I have appointments with them also? If so, how often?	
❖ *If there are other care providers in the practice:* How long have they been in practice? Do I have a choice about whom I see and who delivers the baby?	
❖ What's the rotation schedule?	
❖ How often will I have appointments during my pregnancy?	

Candidate II	Candidate III

	Candidate I
❖ What usually takes place during an appointment?	
❖ What kind of options do I have for prenatal vitamins if the one you prescribe doesn't agree with me?	
❖ Do you recommend childbirth education? If so, do you recommend any classes, methods, or instructors in particular?	
❖ Do you recommend that I also use a labor assistant, or doula, and if so, is there anyone whom you could refer me to?	
❖ How do you feel about husbands or other family members or friends being involved at prenatal exams and during labor and birth?	
❖ What prenatal tests do you routinely recommend?	
❖ How do you feel about patients declining genetic screening tests if they are sure they will keep their babies regardless of the results? What about declining glucose tolerance tests if there aren't any predisposing risk factors?	
❖ What symptoms would you consider serious enough that I should contact you day or night?	
❖ What kind of pain relief options will I have during labor?	

Candidate II	Candidate III

	Candidate I
❖ Are nondrug pain relief options, such as a birthing tub, available? How many of your deliveries last year were nonmedicated births?	
❖ What is your cesarean section rate? What is the rate at the facilities where you deliver?	
❖ What's the ratio of labor and delivery nurses to patients at the facilities where you deliver?	
❖ Do these facilities have obstetrical anesthesiologists on call 24 hours a day?	
❖ If I decide to have an epidural, do you suggest that I consult with the anesthesiologist before labor?	
❖ What are your standing orders for your patients who have been admitted and are in labor?	
❖ Do you routinely order amniotomies (the artificial breaking of a mother's bag of waters)?	
❖ Do you order routine enemas or pubic shaving? What about Pitocin® or other drugs to hasten labor? What about IVs or heparin locks?	
❖ When do you usually try to arrive during a mother's birthing process?	
❖ What do you think about elective cesarean sections?	

Candidate II	Candidate III

	Candidate I
❖ What percentage of your patients have instrumental deliveries (vacuum extraction or forceps)?	
❖ What percentage of your patients are given an episiotomy? *A rate of more than 10 percent is considered excessive.*	
❖ Will you perform intermittent fetal monitoring for my baby, or will I be hooked up to an electronic fetal monitor (EFM) during my labor? How much freedom of movement will an EFM give me?	
❖ What is your policy when labor stalls or when dilation is slow? Are there time limits?	
❖ What are your protocols for fetal distress?	
❖ How do you feel about written birth plans?	
❖ Do you do a postpartum home visit?	
❖ Are there any fees that my health insurance doesn't cover that I should be aware of?	
❖ Other questions and notes:	

Candidate II	Candidate III

Medical History Questions

Your healthcare provider will want to be aware of any conditions that might affect your pregnancy or your baby. Toward that end, during your first prenatal appointment, you'll be asked lots of questions about your own medical history, as well as that of your baby's father and both of your families.

We've provided a sample questionnaire to help you gather information in advance. Not all care providers ask the same questions. Some questions can feel very personal. If you are uncomfortable writing down the answers to any of them, you can leave those spaces blank and ask your care provider if the information is necessary.

Basic Personal Information

❖ Date of birth: _____

❖ Pre-pregnancy weight: _____

❖ Ethnicity: _____

❖ Insurance plan and membership number: _____

_____

❖ Social Security number: _____

❖ Marital status: _____

❖ What was the date of your last menstrual period? _____

❖ At what age did your periods begin? _____

❖ How long do your periods typically last? _____

How often do they occur? _____

❖ Do you have bleeding between periods? _____

❖ What kind of contraceptives have you used in the past year? _____

_____

❖ Have you ever been tested or treated for infertility? _____

Medications

❖ List all of the medications you've taken in the past month, including medicated skin creams, suppositories, and over-the-counter medicines, as well as any vitamins and herbal or dietary supplements:

_____

_____

_____

_____

_____

❖ List any known drug allergies or reactions: _____

_____

_____

_____

_____

Work

❖ If you work outside the home, what kind of work do you do? _____

❖ Is your job physically challenging, requiring heavy lifting or lots of standing? _____

❖ Do you work with chemicals or radiation? _____

❖ Do you work in a day-care or medical facility? _____

❖ How would you rate your daily stress level? _____

Immunizations

❖ When was your last tetanus shot? _____

❖ Have you had a flu or pneumonia vaccine? _____

Illnesses/Conditions/Surgeries

❖ Have you had any illnesses as a child or as an adult that required a hospital stay?

_____

_____

❖ Have you had any in- or outpatient surgeries? _____

_____

_____

❖ Have you had any of the following symptoms or conditions?

Abdominal pain _____

Abnormal Pap smear? If so, when, and what was the method of treatment? ____

_____

Allergies, in the form of eye irritation, nasal congestion, or skin rashes _____

_____

Anemia _____

Arm or leg pain _____

Arthritis _____

Asthma _____

Bladder conditions _____

Blood clots _____

Bowel problems _____

Burning or pain while urinating _____

Cancer _____

Chest pain or pressure _____

Chlamydia _____

Chronic fatigue _____

Depression _____

Diabetes (type I or II) _____

Eating disorder _____

Eye injury or eye condition _____

    Last eye exam: _____

Fainting or dizziness _____

Food allergies

Gallbladder problems

Genital warts

Gonorrhea

Head injury

Hearing or ear problems

Heart disease

Heart murmur

Hemorrhoids

Herpes

High blood pressure or hypertension

High cholesterol or high triglycerides

Joint pain

Kidney inflammation

Lactose intolerance

Liver conditions, such as jaundice, hepatitis, or cirrhosis

Migraines or frequent headaches

Nosebleeds

Numbness or tingling

Ovarian cysts

Rapid or irregular heartbeat or palpitations

Seizures

Sexual difficulty/discomfort

Shortness of breath

Sickle-cell anemia or sickle-cell trait

Sinus problems or infections

Syphilis

Thyroid problems

Unexplained weight gain

Unexplained weight loss

Uterine fibroids

Varicose veins

❖ Have you had any other symptoms or conditions? _____

_____

_____

_____

_____

Personal Habits/Lifestyle

❖ Do you smoke cigarettes, pipes, or cigars? If so, how many a day? _____

At what age did you start smoking? _____

❖ Does anyone in your home smoke? _____

❖ Do you drink alcoholic beverages? If so, how many drinks per week, typically? ___

_____

❖ Have you used any recreational drugs in the past year? _____

❖ Have you taken any drugs (prescription, over-the-counter, or recreational) since you became pregnant? _____

❖ Have you ever been threatened or physically hurt by anyone? _____

_____

❖ How is your relationship with your partner? _____

❖ Have you ever received psychiatric treatment? _____

❖ How much caffeinated coffee, tea, and/or soda do you drink daily? _____

❖ What's your daily calcium intake? _____

❖ How often do you exercise? _____

❖ What type of exercise do you do? _____

❖ Do you have any other concerns you'd like to discuss? _____

_____

_____

_____

_____

Other Pregnancies

❖ How many biological children do you have?

❖ What are their ages?

❖ What were their birth weights?

❖ How many times have you been pregnant, not including this instance?

❖ Have you had any miscarriages or stillbirths? If so, how far along were you?

Past Pregnancy Complications

❖ Have you had any of the following?

Bleeding after the twelfth week of pregnancy

Cerclage

Cesarean section

Gestational diabetes

Placental abruption

Placenta previa

Postpartum depression for longer than two weeks

Preeclampsia or toxemia

Preterm labor

Family History

Your Father

❖ Age if living, or age at death:

❖ If deceased, cause of death:

❖ Has he ever had any of the following?

Cancer

Any cardiovascular conditions, such as hypertension, heart disease, heart attack, or stroke

Diabetes (type I or II)

Kidney disease

Thyroid condition

Any other chronic health conditions: _____

_____

_____

_____

Your Mother

❖ Age if living, or age at death: _____

❖ If deceased, cause of death: _____

❖ Has she ever had any of the following?

Cancer _____

Any cardiovascular conditions, such as hypertension, heart disease, heart attack, or stroke _____

Cesarean section _____

Depression or postpartum depression for longer than two weeks _____

Diabetes (type I, type II, or gestational) _____

Endometriosis _____

Kidney disease _____

Placental abruption _____

Preeclampsia or eclampsia _____

Premature infants, or babies weighing less than 5.5 pounds at birth _____

Thyroid condition _____

Uterine fibroids _____

Any other chronic health conditions: _____

_____

_____

Any other health issues during any of her pregnancies: _____

_____

_____

Did she ever take DES (diethylstilbestrol)? _____

Your Sibling(s)

❖ Age(s): _____

❖ If any are deceased, cause of death: _____

❖ Have any of your siblings ever had any of the following?

Cancer _____

Any cardiovascular conditions, such as hypertension, heart disease, heart attack, or stroke _____

Cesarean section _____

Depression or postpartum depression for longer than two weeks ___

Diabetes (type I, type II, or gestational) _____

Endometriosis _____

Kidney disease _____

Placental abruption _____

Preeclampsia or eclampsia _____

Premature infants, or babies weighing less than 5.5 pounds at birth _

Thyroid condition _____

Uterine fibroids _____

Any other chronic health conditions: _____

_____

_____

_____

Any other health issues during pregnancy: _____

_____

_____

_____

All Relatives

❖ Was anyone in your family or in your baby's father's family born with any genetic conditions, such as:

Cystic fibrosis _____

Down syndrome _____

Hemophilia _____

Huntington's chorea

Mental retardation

Muscular dystrophy

Phenylketonuria (PKU)

Sickle-cell anemia

Tay-Sachs disease

Thalassemia

Any other genetic conditions:

Prenatal Appointments

Date: _____   Time: _____

Questions to ask my care provider:

Responses:

Other information and notes:

Prenatal Appointments

Date: _____   **Time:** _____

Questions to ask my care provider:

Responses:

Other information and notes:

Prenatal Appointments

Date: _____   Time: _____

Questions to ask my care provider:

Responses:

Other information and notes:

Prenatal Appointments

Date: _____   **Time:** _____

Questions to ask my care provider:

Responses:

Other information and notes:

Prenatal Appointments

Date: _____   Time: _____

Questions to ask my care provider:

Responses:

Other information and notes:

Prenatal Appointments

Date: _____   Time: _____

Questions to ask my care provider:

Responses:

Other information and notes:

Prenatal Appointments

Date: _____   **Time:** _____

Questions to ask my care provider:

Responses:

Other information and notes:

Prenatal Appointments

Date: _____   Time: _____

Questions to ask my care provider:

Responses:

Other information and notes:

Prenatal Appointments

Date: _____   **Time:** _____

Questions to ask my care provider:

Responses:

Other information and notes:

Prenatal Appointments

Date: _____   Time: _____

Questions to ask my care provider:

Responses:

Other information and notes:

Prenatal Appointments

Date: _____   Time: _____

Questions to ask my care provider:

Responses:

Other information and notes:

Prenatal Appointments

Date: _____   **Time:** _____

Questions to ask my care provider:

Responses:

Other information and notes:

Prenatal Appointments

Date: _____   Time: _____

Questions to ask my care provider:

Responses:

Other information and notes:

Prenatal Appointments

Date: _____   Time: _____

Questions to ask my care provider:

Responses:

Other information and notes:

Prenatal Appointments

Date: _____   **Time:** _____

Questions to ask my care provider:

Responses:

Other information and notes:

Diagnostic and Screening Tests

Type: _____ **Date:** _____

Name and number of testing facility:

Date result will be available and whom to call:

Notes:

Type: _____ **Date:** _____

Name and number of testing facility:

Date result will be available and whom to call:

Notes:

Diagnostic and Screening Tests

Type: _____   Date: _____

Name and number of testing facility:

Date result will be available and whom to call:

Notes:

Type: _____   Date: _____

Name and number of testing facility:

Date result will be available and whom to call:

Notes:

Diagnostic and Screening Tests

Type: _____   Date: _____

Name and number of testing facility:

Date result will be available and whom to call:

Notes:

Type: _____   Date: _____

Name and number of testing facility:

Date result will be available and whom to call:

Notes:

Diagnostic and Screening Tests

Type: _____ Date: _____

Name and number of testing facility:

Date result will be available and whom to call:

Notes:

Type: _____ Date: _____

Name and number of testing facility:

Date result will be available and whom to call:

Notes:

Diagnostic and Screening Tests

Type: _____ Date: _____

Name and number of testing facility:

Date result will be available and whom to call:

Notes:

Type: _____ Date: _____

Name and number of testing facility:

Date result will be available and whom to call:

Notes:

Postpartum Exam

Date: _____   **Time:** _____

Following are some questions you may want to ask:

Is it okay for me to drive? _____

Can I resume exercising? _____

If so, what kind of exercises can I do? _____

_____

Can I resume sexual activity? _____

Are my stitches healed? Can I take hot baths? _____

Can you recommend birth control options? _____

_____

Other questions to ask:

_____

_____

_____

_____

Other information and notes:

_____

_____

_____

_____

_____

_____

Finding a Pediatrician

While it is important for you and your partner to meet the doctor and her staff in person when considering a pediatrician for your baby, there are some practical questions that you can ask ahead of time over the phone. Thus, the following interview has been divided into two sections: The first part contains questions you may want to ask a staff member before going into the office to meet with the pediatrician; the second part contains questions for an in-person conversation with the doctor.

	Pediatrician/Practice I
Pediatrician/practice:	
Address:	
Phone:	
Fax:	
Questions for the receptionist via phone:	
❖ Hello, I'm expecting and due on (*date*). Is Dr. (*name*) accepting new patients?	
❖ *If the doctor isn't accepting new patients:* Can you recommend another doctor?	
❖ Do you accept my health insurance?	
❖ What hospital(s) does the doctor have privileges with?	
❖ Is a bio or profile of the doctor available?	
❖ Where exactly is the office located?	
❖ What are the regular office hours?	

Pediatrician/Practice II	Pediatrician/Practice III

	Pediatrician/Practice I
❖ Do you have more than one office, and if so, how is the doctor's time divided between them?	
❖ Do you have a regularly scheduled time when parents can call with nonemergency medical questions?	
❖ How many patients does the doctor see on a typical day?	
❖ How long does the doctor usually spend with each patient during a routine visit?	
❖ How far in advance do you recommend making appointments?	
❖ On average, how long do people with appointments sit in the waiting room before seeing the doctor?	
❖ Do you have a separate waiting room for sick children?	
❖ Do you have laboratory facilities on-site?	
❖ Can you provide vision and hearing screenings on-site?	
❖ Do you charge for canceled or missed appointments or for filling out paperwork?	
❖ Can I schedule a consultation with the doctor?	
Questions to ask the pediatrician:	
❖ How long have you been in practice?	
❖ Where did you go to school?	
❖ Do you have any special training or certifications?	

Pediatrician/Practice II	Pediatrician/Practice III

	Pediatrician/Practice I
❖ Are you the only person we'll see each time we bring our baby in, or is there an assistant or another physician who will also be providing medical care?	
❖ *If there are other doctors or nurses in the practice:* What sort of experience do the other care providers have?	
❖ Who provides backup for you during evenings and weekends?	
❖ What do you suggest we do if there is an emergency during office hours? What about when the office is closed?	
❖ How soon after the baby is born can you examine him/her? Do you make visits to the hospital where I'm delivering? If not, when should we call to make our baby's first appointment?	
❖ How quickly are you usually able to return telephone calls?	
❖ What are your opinions regarding: Breastfeeding? Circumcision? Co-sleeping versus crib sleeping? Pacifier use? My lifestyle: occupation, marital status and living situation, age, religious or dietary practices? The hospital where I plan to deliver? My obstetrician?	

Pediatrician/Practice II	Pediatrician/Practice III

	Pediatrician/Practice I
❖ How many routine visits will we need to schedule during the first year?	
❖ What is your preferred immunization schedule for infants? Can you give me some literature about which vaccines will be needed and when and what the possible side effects are?	
❖ How do you feel about parents seeking a second opinion on medical decisions?	
❖ *If you plan to breastfeed:* Can you refer me to a lactation consultant, or do you have one on staff who will be available to visit me at the hospital/birth center and after I go home?	
❖ What services can you offer me if we discover that I have a high-risk pregnancy?	
❖ Do you have any suggestions regarding what I should or should not be doing during the last months of my pregnancy?	
❖ Other questions and information:	

Pediatrician/Practice II	Pediatrician/Practice III

Questions to Ask a Childbirth Educator

Following are some questions you may want to ask when you're looking into childbirth classes.

	Childbirth Educator I
Class:	
Address:	
Phone:	
Name of instructor:	
❖ How long does the course last?	
❖ Do you offer shorter (or longer) versions?	
❖ Do I need to have a birth partner to attend?	
❖ About how many people are in each class?	
❖ How would you describe the method that the class teaches?	
❖ What can I expect to learn?	
❖ What are the available class dates and times?	
❖ What is the fee?	

Childbirth Educator II	Childbirth Educator III

	Childbirth Educator I
❖ Is any portion of the fee covered by my health insurance policy?	
❖ Do you have any preferred books and videos and/or a list of recommended Web sites?	
❖ Other questions and information:	
❖ Directions to class:	

Childbirth Educator II	Childbirth Educator III

Questions to Ask a Labor Assistant (Doula)

Following are some questions you may want to ask when meeting with labor assistants.

	Labor Assistant I
Name:	
Address:	
Phone:	
❖ How many births have you attended?	
❖ What type of childbirth classes do you recommend? *Some doulas may require that you take certain classes.*	
❖ Will you be available in the two weeks before and the two weeks after my due date?	
❖ Do you also offer postpartum support visits? If not, can you recommend someone who does?	
❖ What are your fees?	
❖ At what point during labor should I call you?	
❖ Would you be available if I go into active labor in the middle of the night?	
❖ Have you worked with my care provider before? If you have, what were your impressions?	
❖ Have you supported deliveries in the healthcare facility where I plan to have my baby? If so, how do you feel about that facility?	

Labor Assistant II	Labor Assistant III

	Labor Assistant I
❖ What are your feelings about the use of pain relief medication during labor?	
❖ How will my experience be different if I have an epidural versus a nonmedicated labor?	
❖ Please describe the relaxation techniques you use.	
❖ What do you think about women eating, drinking, and getting out of bed during labor?	
❖ Do you usually bring accessories, like a birth ball, massaging foot roller, aromatherapy oils, or other relaxation devices?	
❖ How would you help me if I have an induction? A cesarean section?	
❖ Are you also a licensed massage therapist?	
❖ Other questions and information:	
References	
❖ Name: ❖ Phone: ❖ Questions: ❖ Comments:	

Labor Assistant II	Labor Assistant III

	Labor Assistant I
❖ Name: ❖ Phone: ❖ Questions: ❖ Comments:	
❖ Name: ❖ Phone: ❖ Questions: ❖ Comments:	
❖ Name: ❖ Phone: ❖ Questions: ❖ Comments:	

Labor Assistant II	Labor Assistant III

Creating Your Birth Plan

The best approach when creating a birth plan is to treat it more as a series of desires and wishes than rules hewn in stone. It's important to discuss everything with your healthcare provider, ask him what kind of experience you can reasonably expect to have, and make sure you fully understand all of the factors involved with your options. Following are some topics to consider.

Your Strategy for Pain Management

❖ Do you want a nonmedicated birth? If so, do you want the opportunity to:
   – use a tub or shower? _____
   _____
   – walk around? _____
   _____
   – use the coaching services of a labor assistant or doula? _____
   _____
   – have a specific ambience, such as dimmed lights or soft music? _____
   _____
   – use labor accessories, such as a birth ball, birthing stool, or beanbag? ___
   _____
   – practice acupressure, acupuncture, or guided relaxation techniques? _____
   _____

❖ Do you want a medicated birth? If so, do you want to be offered:
   – an epidural as soon as possible? _____
   _____
   – narcotics, sedatives, and/or other nonepidural pain medications? _____
   _____

❖ Do you want to start with a nonmedicated delivery but be offered the option of having an epidural or other pain medications as labor progresses, should you decide that you want them? _____

❖ Or do you want your care provider to help suggest what might work best for you? _____
_____

❖ Are you not sure yet, and want to decide once you get to the hospital? *You should still make sure to discuss all of the options in detail with your healthcare provider ahead of time.*

Your Hospital Experience

❖ Do you have any allergies or conditions that could affect labor, birth, or your use of pain-relieving medications?

❖ Do you have any psychological conditions or specific fears or worries that the hospital staff should know about?

❖ What levels of intervention are you comfortable with?

❖ Do you mind being given a routine IV for fluids?

❖ Will you be shaved or given an enema?

❖ Are there interventions you want to avoid for religious reasons, such as blood transfusions?

❖ If you've previously had a cesarean delivery, do you want the opportunity to deliver vaginally this time? *Many hospitals prohibit this, so it's important to discuss this issue with your care provider in advance.*

❖ What's the hospital's policy on continuous electronic fetal monitoring? Can you have intermittent monitoring instead?

❖ Can you decline drugs to have your contractions strengthened?

❖ Does the hospital allow you to eat and/or drink while you're in labor?

❖ Who do you want to have in the room with you?

❖ Who do you want kept out?

❖ Is there a specific procedure that you're trying to avoid, such as an amniotomy, an episiotomy, or a cesarean section?

❖ Is your hospital a teaching hospital? If so, do you mind being tended to or visited by medical residents?

Delivery
❖ How do you want to participate in the birth? Do you want to:
  – be told when to rest and when to push, or push as you feel the urge?

  – touch the baby's head as it crowns?

  – watch the birth in a mirror?

  – have someone record baby's delivery on video or have it photographed?

  – have your partner catch the baby or cut the umbilical cord?

  – have the baby placed on your chest immediately after delivery or wait until the baby has been cleaned and weighed?

  – have newborn procedures such as weighing and fingerprinting performed in the room or in the nursery?

❖ If a cesarean is necessary:
   – will you be awake?
   _____

   – will your partner be allowed in the room?
   _____

   – do you want the drape removed when it's time for the baby to be lifted out?
   _____

Recovery

❖ Do you plan to breastfeed? If so, is there a lactation consultant on staff? If the baby has to go to the NICU, will the hospital help you pump milk?
_____
_____

❖ Do you want to be offered pain medication after birth?
_____

❖ How soon after delivery will your care provider check up on you?
❖ Will the recovery room have a place for your partner to sleep?
❖ Will your recovery room be private?
❖ Will you be able to make room requests (e.g., requesting a room near the nurse's station or one with a view)?
❖ Do you want the baby to be in your room around the clock, only when you're awake, or just for feedings?
❖ Do you plan to have your son circumcised in the hospital? If so, who will perform the procedure? Do you have specific pain relief preferences for your son (e.g., a dorsal nerve block or a topical anesthetic)?
_____
_____

❖ How long will you stay in the hospital/birthing center after a normal birth? What about after a cesarean delivery? Do you want to stay in the hospital/birth center for as long as possible, or check out as quickly as you can?
_____
_____

PART THREE

Baby

Steps

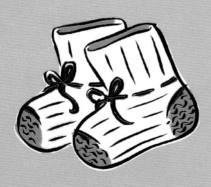

The Baby Shower and Registry

Baby showers are typically held anywhere from Week 34 to Week 36 and are traditionally hosted by a close friend or relative other than the expectant mom's sibling or mother. While they used to be all-female affairs, some now include dads-to-be and male friends, too. If you're expecting twins or multiples, it's better that the shower take place earlier than the last month of your pregnancy, since you may go into labor sooner than expected or end up with doctor's orders for bed rest.

Here are some practical tips for your baby gift registry and shower:

❖ Take stock of what you have and what you'll need before you register.

❖ Select at least one national retail chain to register with so that friends and family from out of state will be able to purchase gifts from your wish list.

❖ Choose items in a variety of price ranges so that all of your friends and relatives can find items on your registry within their budgets.

❖ Test out items in the store, and choose carefully. While you can always return stuff, it's better to get what you want the first time around!

❖ Venture out of the baby department. Consider adding towels, washcloths, clothes hampers, unscented detergent, and other household goods. You'll need that stuff, too.

❖ Try to be a good sport at the shower—even if your hostess insists on games like "guess the pregnant lady's weight."

❖ Be sure to record what you get from everyone and send thank-you notes (you can use the space provided on page 166).

❖ Don't forget to thank the hostess with flowers and a note afterward.

❖ Save gift receipts in an envelope, and put the envelope somewhere safe and easy to find. You may not realize you need to return something until after the baby is born.

❖ Fill out and send in product registration cards so that you'll be notified in the event of a recall.

Get Ready, Get Set, Go!

You've got a lot to accomplish before your baby arrives! There are clothes and supplies to buy, steps to take to prepare for your baby's delivery, and things you can do to help your household run a bit more smoothly after your baby is born. In the last few weeks of your pregnancy, you'll probably start to feel rather heavy and uncomfortable, so plan to do as much as you can before then.

To assist you with the prep work, there are checklists of maternity wear and baby gear. The latter includes not only basic necessities, but also items you may find helpful to have on hand. Keep in mind that access to a well-functioning washing machine and dryer will be useful.

Another important thing you can do to prepare for your baby's arrival is to tour the hospital or birth center where you'll deliver. Scoping out the place ahead of time will make you more comfortable in your surroundings on the big day; plus, you can often use your time there to take care of some admission procedures in advance so that there's less to do when you go into labor. Most hospitals and birth centers have regular tours scheduled once or twice a week; you'll need to call ahead to make an appointment. When you head to the hospital or birth center for your tour, take the opportunity to map out the best routes there; it is also helpful to determine the parking situation for you and your visitors, as well as to check out nearby options for takeout food in case hospital food turns out to be unappetizing. See the section beginning on page 169 for some things you can do and ask to help make the tour as useful as possible.

If you know you'll need childcare arrangements after the baby is born, you'll probably want to get this lined up while you're still pregnant. Your second trimester is not too early to start looking for an infant caregiver or a childcare center that accepts babies, as the process can take a while and good professionals and places tend to get booked up quickly. In this chapter, you'll find some questions you might want to ask when trying to determine which professional or facility is the best fit for you and your baby (see the sections beginning on pages 176 and 182).

Outfitting Yourself

While you may need to purchase some items earlier, it's best to do your serious shopping for maternity clothes around Week 20 to get the most wear out of them (before then, you may be able to get by with pants that are oversized or have an elastic waistband). Not only is Week 20 the halfway point of your pregnancy, but the size you are then is roughly the size you'll be for about six weeks postpartum. Buy shirts, pants, and dresses that are the right length but still give you space to grow in the hips, stomach, and chest. Keep in mind that there's probably no need to buy an expensive brand-new wardrobe. You can also get clothes on auction Web sites, at thrift and discount stores, and at consignment shops. And don't forget friends and relatives, who may be only too happy to lend or give you maternity wear they no longer need.

Your Shopping Checklist

- [ ] Jeans or pants with expandable panels
- [ ] Maternity shirts long enough to cover the elastic panels on maternity pants (pick button-down shirts and/or stretchy knits if you're planning to breastfeed)
- [ ] One or two maternity dresses for formal occasions
- [ ] At least a week's worth of maternity underwear (bikini styles tend to be the most versatile)
- [ ] A supportive bra or two in natural fabrics, nursing-style if you plan to breastfeed (note that your breasts and rib cage will continue to expand until you give birth, so it's a good idea to buy only one or two bras at a time)
- [ ] Maternity bathing suit, if you swim
- [ ] Flat-soled slip-on shoes (you may go up as much as a full size from your pre-pregnancy days)
- [ ] Slipper socks with nonslip treads
- [ ] Maternity hose, if you wear stockings to work
- [ ] Roomy bathrobe (especially useful during your time at the birthing facility and during postpartum weeks)
- [ ] Sunscreen and a wide-brimmed hat for use outdoors to help minimize the effects of pregnancy-related skin discoloration
- [ ] Box of nursing pads (even if you plan to bottle-feed)

Baby's Gear

The following checklists contain basic baby items that you'll need, as well as ones that you may find helpful to have. It is important to get the safest, most durable, and most baby-friendly products, so do thorough research before purchasing or registering for anything.

The three most important pieces of baby equipment you'll need are a crib, a mattress, and a car seat designed for infants. For maximum safety you should definitely buy your baby's crib mattress and car seat new. And remember, as with other baby products, there are a host of specific safety issues to consider and look into, so be sure to do your homework.

Car seats are classified by the weight of their passengers. Weight requirements are usually printed on a tag attached to the seat and on the side of the seat's packaging.

Safe installation requires studying two sources: the instructions that come with the car seat and the owner's manual for your car. The latter will show you how to use the seat-belts or anchors in your car's backseat and will also warn you about unsafe seat positions, such as in front of airbags and armrests. Install your baby's car seat well in advance of your due date (especially if you're expecting multiples), and make an appointment to have your installation inspected by a representative of your local police or fire department.

Nursery Equipment & Supplies

Necessities:

- [ ] Chest of drawers, open shelf, or some other way to store and organize baby clothes and supplies
- [ ] Crib
- [ ] Crib mattress
- [ ] Fitted crib sheets
- [ ] Crib bumper
- [ ] Diaper pail

Nice to have, but optional:

- [ ] Changing table and changing pad (ideally one for each floor of the house)
- [ ] Crib mattress pad
- [ ] Crib mobile

☐ Mesh crib tent (if you have cats, to keep them out of baby's sleeping area)
☐ Rocking chair or glider with a footstool
☐ Waterproof pads to protect your clothes from spit-up
☐ Night light

Baby's Clothes

Necessities:

☐ Outfit for baby to wear home from hospital/birth center
☐ Onesies (one-piece garments that cover baby's top and bottom and snap at the crotch) for daily use (expect to use two or three a day)
☐ Socks or booties
☐ Baby sweaters and a bunting for winter
☐ Sleep sac or footed sleepers for winter
☐ Hats (to protect against sun in warm weather or to keep warm in cold weather)

Nice to have, but optional:

☐ Dressier outfits for special occasions

Travel Gear

Necessities:

☐ Infant-only or "convertible" (infant-to-toddler) car seat
☐ Diaper bag or an ordinary backpack with lots of roomy compartments
☐ Portable changing pad
☐ Soft carrier or sling
☐ Reclining stroller

Nice to have, but optional:

☐ Car window shades
☐ Jog stroller
☐ Portable crib
☐ Sheets for portable crib
☐ Activity bar for stroller

Feeding Baby

Necessities:

☐ Bibs (reusable or disposable)

☐ Bottle brush

☐ Nipple brush

☐ Three or four bottles (don't buy a lot until you find out what style you and your baby prefer)

☐ Several newborn-size silicone nipples

If you plan to bottle-feed:

☐ Small container of formula (ask the pediatrician you select for your baby what his brand preference is, and wait to see how your baby tolerates the brand before stocking up)

Nice for breastfeeding, but optional:

☐ Breastfeeding pillow, such as the Boppy® (made by the Boppy Company)

☐ Breast pump

☐ Milk storage bottles

☐ Nipple cream

☐ Nursing shirts

Nice for bottle-feeding, but optional:

☐ Nipple basket for dishwasher

☐ Microwave sterilizer for bottles, nipples, and pacifiers

Bathing and Caring for Baby

Necessities:

☐ Antibiotic ointment

☐ Baby wipes

☐ Diaper rash cream

☐ Baby-strength acetaminophen

☐ Medicine dropper

☐ Baby nail clippers

☐ Nasal aspirator (suction bulb) to clear your baby's nose in case of congestion

☐ Newborn-size diapers (expect to use six to eight a day)
☐ Receiving blanket(s), for swaddling and protecting clothes from spit-up
☐ Saline nose drops
☐ Thermometer (ask your pediatrician what type he recommends)
☐ Washcloths or cloth diapers for clean-up
☐ Petroleum jelly
☐ Baby soap and tearless baby shampoo

Nice to have, but optional:

☐ Baby hairbrush and comb
☐ Hooded bath towel
☐ Baby bathtub

Miscellaneous

Nice to have, but optional:

☐ Audio or video monitor
☐ Camera or camcorder
☐ Pacifiers
☐ Play gym
☐ Rattles
☐ Safety gates
☐ Scrapbook, photo boxes, and photo albums
☐ Stationary exerciser and/or bouncer seat
☐ Automatic baby swing
☐ Teether

My Registry Information

Store/Web site:

Address:

Phone: Password:

Store/Web site:

Address:

Phone: Password:

Store/Web site:

Address:

Phone: Password:

Store/Web site:

Address:

Phone: Password:

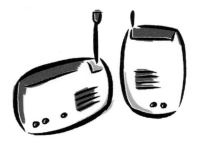

Gift Tracker

Giver	Present	Thank-you mailed
		☐
		☐
		☐
		☐
		☐
		☐
		☐
		☐
		☐
		☐
		☐
		☐
		☐
		☐
		☐
		☐
		☐

Gift Tracker

Giver	Present	Thank-you mailed
		☐
		☐
		☐
		☐
		☐
		☐
		☐
		☐
		☐
		☐
		☐
		☐
		☐
		☐
		☐
		☐
		☐
		☐

Gift Tracker

Giver	Present	Thank-you mailed
		☐
		☐
		☐
		☐
		☐
		☐
		☐
		☐
		☐
		☐
		☐
		☐
		☐
		☐
		☐
		☐
		☐
		☐

Your Birthing Facility Tour

To make your tour as productive and informative as possible, you may wish to make note of the following information.

❖ How long it takes to get there: _____

❖ The quickest route: _____

_____

_____

_____

_____

_____

❖ Alternate routes (in case of traffic jams or construction): _____

_____

_____

_____

_____

_____

_____

_____

❖ Locations of the closest convenience stores, delis, and restaurants offering takeout (in case the facility's food is unappealing or available only during certain hours):

_____

_____

❖ Personal observations regarding the birthing suites and recovery rooms:

_____

_____

_____

Tour Questions

Following are some questions that may be useful to ask during your tour of the birthing facility.

❖ Where should we park when I come to be admitted? Can we have our parking passes validated?

❖ Where should I go to be admitted?

❖ Is there a different procedure if I arrive after hours?

❖ Can I complete pre-admission forms before I leave today or take them home to fill out in advance, so I won't have to do it when I'm in labor?

❖ Will I be sharing my room with another mother? If so, how can I arrange for a private room instead?

❖ How many visitors can I have in my room and in the waiting room—during birth and after?

❖ What are regular visiting hours?

❖ What is the procedure for visitors?

❖ Are there age restrictions for visitors?

❖ Do visitors need to bring identification? What kind of security measures are in place to keep unauthorized people out of the maternity ward?

❖ What are your feelings about pre-written birth plans? Should I bring a copy of mine for my file when I arrive in labor?

❖ Does your birthing facility have written policies it follows for all laboring patients? Are they open for viewing by potential patients?

❖ What is this facility's policy about eating or drinking during labor?

❖ Where is the hospital cafeteria located?
❖ How many babies are born here each year?
❖ What is the ratio of certified labor and delivery nurses to patients?
❖ Is there a maximum number of patients that an individual nurse can be assigned to at one time?
❖ Do you have special birthing rooms that allow a mother to labor and give birth in the same place? Do all mothers get to give birth in those rooms? If not, where do labor and delivery occur?

❖ *If the facility is a teaching hospital or affiliated with one:* Will medical students and residents be involved in my care? If so, will the person who supervises them be in attendance at all times? Do I have the right to refuse treatment from a physician-in-training? How do I request that?

❖ What do you suggest I do if I find myself disagreeing with a procedure recommended by a healthcare provider during labor? Can I request a second opinion? Whom should I turn to in the facility to get that opinion?

❖ Is there a lactation consultant on your staff? How do I obtain her services?

❖ What are typical nursing shifts?
❖ Will my baby be able to nurse immediately after birth?

❖ What services does the hospital nursery offer mothers? Do you offer the option of around-the-clock rooming-in for babies?

_____

_____

❖ Where is the nursery?

❖ Does the birthing wing have the services of obstetrical anesthesiologists? Are they available 24/7? Will I be able to discuss my pain relief preferences and any special conditions with such a professional before I go into labor? How do I make an appointment for a consultation?

_____

_____

_____

_____

❖ What is this facility's policy on continuous electronic fetal monitoring (EFM)? Is intermittent monitoring available upon request?

_____

_____

❖ If I have my labor induced or augmented, will I be able to control the level of medication?

_____

❖ What is the facility's C-section rate?

❖ What is the hospital's procedure if I need a cesarean? May I see the area where cesareans are performed? Where will I be moved for recovery? Will my partner be allowed in the operating room with me?

_____

_____

_____

_____

❖ What routine tests, vaccinations, medications, and/or procedures will be given/done to my baby before being released from this facility?

_____

_____

❖ Where are circumcisions performed, and who performs them?

❖ Does the hospital have a policy about the pain medications used for babies during circumcision?

❖ May I have copies of the "informed consent" forms you require for special labor and delivery situations so that I can read them in advance?

❖ How long will I be allowed to stay here after a normal birth? After a cesarean delivery?

❖ What care facilities do you offer newborns with special needs? Do you have a neonatal intensive care unit (NICU)? If not, how far away is the nearest NICU, and how are babies transferred? What are the NICU's visiting policies?

❖ What will I need to do in order to enter the NICU to visit my baby? Would you recommend we take a look at the NICU and speak with someone there?

❖ *If you're planning to breastfeed:* If the baby has to go to the NICU, will I be furnished with a breast pump and will someone be available to instruct me how to use it?

❖ Other questions and information:

Packing for the Big Day

While there are some items that you won't be able to pack until it's almost time to be on your way to the birthing facility, you'll want to have as much as possible ready to go ahead of time.

Don't forget these items:

☐ Health insurance card

☐ Baby car seat, installed facing rearward in your car and in accordance with the instructions that came with the car seat and the directions in your vehicle owner's manual

☐ Outfit for your baby to wear home

☐ Cell phone and charger (note that you may need to leave it off until you are in a recovery room, and some hospitals ban their use inside the building completely, as their signals can interfere with certain types of monitoring equipment)

☐ Deodorant

☐ Brush and/or comb

☐ Toothbrush

☐ Toothpaste

☐ Maternity underwear (two or three pairs; the hospital may supply disposables, but you should bring some just in case)

☐ Socks (the kind with nonslip soles are best)

☐ Bathrobe and slippers

☐ List of phone numbers of relatives and friends to be notified (space for compiling this information is provided on page 202)

☐ This book

☐ A pre-addressed return packet for your baby's cord blood sample, if you plan to use a cord blood bank

☐ _____

☐ _____

☐ _____

☐ _____

☐ _____

Optional items:

☐ Photocopies of your medical records (including ones from your prior healthcare providers, which you should have already supplied to your current care provider), particularly if you are considered high-risk or have a medical condition that might affect birth or recovery

☐ Personal birth plan

☐ Portable music player and favorite songs

☐ Extra batteries for your music player

☐ Healthy snacks, such as high-protein bars and crackers

☐ Bottled water

☐ Legal-size pad and a pen for recording things you want to remember

☐ Folder for taking home hospital documents

☐ Lightweight blanket for your partner

☐ Makeup (expect to be in a lot of photos!)

☐ Lip balm, hand cream, and/or face cream

☐ Hair clips, hair elastics, and/or a headband

☐ Favorite maternity outfit to wear home (note that you'll be about 10 pounds lighter, so pack accordingly)

☐ Camera

☐ Film or photo card

☐ Extra batteries or charger for camera

☐ Change for vending machines and pay phones

☐ Natural childbirth pain relief supplies, such as a birthing ball or back massage tools

☐ Two-level footstool for supporting your feet as you sit in a chair or on the toilet

☐ Cash for a cab ride to the birthing facility—just in case!

You may wish to bring the following items, though they will be supplied by the hospital:

☐ Pillow (put it in a colored pillowcase so that it won't get confused with hospital bedding)

☐ Nightgown with front openings for nursing (something that you don't mind getting stained)

☐ Disposable breast pads (bring a box)

☐ Heavy-flow sanitary napkins

Questions to Ask Infant Caregivers

Following are questions you may want to ask when meeting with and evaluating potential caregivers for your baby. If you're considering more than three candidates, you can make photocopies of the interview form and keep them in the pocket at the end of this book.

	Caregiver I
Name:	
Phone:	
Agency (if applicable):	
❖ What hours are you available?	
❖ Are you also available evenings and weekends?	
❖ Do you have a driver's license?	
❖ What is your citizenship status?	
❖ What kind of experience do you have?	
❖ How many years of experience do you have caring for children?	
❖ Do you believe in putting babies on a schedule for naps and meals?	
❖ Are you certified in infant CPR? If not, will you take a class if I pay for it?	
❖ How much do you charge?	
❖ Do you also do light housework?	

Caregiver II	Caregiver III

	Caregiver I
❖ Have you been convicted of a felony?	
❖ Would you agree to a background check?	
❖ Do you speak any other languages?	
❖ What kinds of discipline methods do you use with children?	
❖ Have you ever been frustrated with a child you were caring for, and if so, what did you do?	
❖ Are you comfortable with our pets?	
❖ Other questions and/or notes:	
References	
❖ Name: ❖ Phone: ❖ Questions: ❖ Comments:	

Caregiver II	Caregiver III

	Caregiver I
❖ Name: ❖ Phone: ❖ Questions: ❖ Comments:	
❖ Name: ❖ Phone: ❖ Questions: ❖ Comments:	
❖ Name: ❖ Phone: ❖ Questions: ❖ Comments:	

Caregiver II	Caregiver III

Questions to Ask at a Childcare Center

Before you head to a childcare center you're considering, you should also take a look at "Things to Observe at a Childcare Center" on page 192.

	Childcare Center I
Childcare center:	
Address:	
Phone:	
Fax:	
E-mail:	
Web site:	
❖ Are you a licensed facility? What agency licenses you?	
❖ Who owns this facility?	
❖ What age ranges do you accept?	
❖ Do you have space available at the time I plan to return to work? If not, can I get on a waiting list?	
❖ What hours are you open?	
❖ Is your facility closed on certain holidays?	
❖ How much do you charge?	
❖ What credentials do you require of your staff members? Do they have special training in infancy? Do you offer in-service training to your staff?	

Childcare Center II	Childcare Center III

	Childcare Center I
❖ What's the staff-to-baby ratio? *There should be no more than three babies for every staff member.*	
❖ Do you have any employees on standby for when staff members become ill or go on vacation?	
❖ What would the daily routine for my baby be like?	
❖ How do you feel about my calling during the day to check on my baby?	
❖ How do you feel about parents visiting their babies during the day?	
❖ Do you feed babies on a certain schedule or on demand?	
❖ What type of baby bottles do you prefer that I use?	
❖ If I supply breast milk, do you have a place to freeze it or refrigerate it until feeding time? Will you warm it up according to my directions?	
❖ Is your toddler play area separate from your baby area?	
❖ Can I do a half-day or every-other-day arrangement?	
❖ Are there penalties for picking up my child late? If so, what are they?	

Childcare Center II	Childcare Center III

	Childcare Center I
❖ What supplies do I need to provide?	
❖ What are your policies regarding sick children?	
❖ How will I be notified if there's an outbreak of a contagious illness?	
❖ Do you ever close for bad weather? How do you inform parents when that happens?	
❖ Can the staff administer prescribed medications?	
❖ What are your procedures for sanitizing the diaper-changing area and the toys?	
❖ How and where do you dispose of dirty diapers?	
❖ Does each baby have his own crib?	
❖ Do you use a professional cleaning service for crib linens? How often are they changed?	
❖ What medical records do you need for your files?	
❖ Do you have a Web cam that will allow me to check on my baby during the day?	
❖ What security measures do you use to keep unauthorized people out?	
❖ How do you handle disruptive children?	

Childcare Center II	Childcare Center III

	Childcare Center I
❖ At what age do you expect children to be toilet-trained?	
❖ Can you supply the names of three or four parents as references? *See the "References" section that starts below.*	
❖ Other questions and/or notes:	
References	
❖ Name: ❖ Phone: ❖ Questions: ❖ Comments:	
❖ Name: ❖ Phone: ❖ Questions: ❖ Comments:	

Childcare Center II	Childcare Center III

	Childcare Center I
❖ Name: ❖ Phone: ❖ Questions: ❖ Comments:	
❖ Name: ❖ Phone: ❖ Questions: ❖ Comments:	

Childcare Center II	Childcare Center III

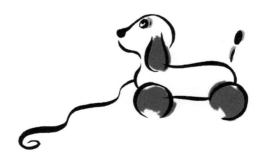

Things to Observe at a Childcare Center

	Childcare Center I
Childcare center:	
❖ Does the atmosphere generally feel warm and affectionate?	
❖ Does the center appear clean and well lit?	
❖ What kinds of stimulation activities are used with babies when they are awake?	
❖ How quickly are crying babies comforted? How does the staff relate to babies who are unhappy?	
❖ Where do sick children wait until they can be picked up?	
❖ What are the sanitizing procedures for the diaper-changing area and for toys?	
❖ Does the staff-to-child ratio seem sufficient?	
❖ Do babies get an opportunity to go outside?	
❖ Other observations:	

Childcare Center II	Childcare Center III

Getting Your House in Order

Following are some household items that you may want to stock up on before your baby arrives to cut down on shopping later.

Food/Drink

- [ ] Bottled water and beverages
- [ ] Canned goods
- [ ] Coffee
- [ ] Flour
- [ ] Frozen foods
- [ ] Pasta
- [ ] Rice
- [ ] Salt
- [ ] Sugar
- [ ] _____
- [ ] _____
- [ ] _____
- [ ] _____
- [ ] _____
- [ ] _____
- [ ] _____
- [ ] _____

General Household Supplies

- [ ] Batteries in various sizes
- [ ] Cleaning supplies (the more labor-saving, the better)
- [ ] Coffee filters
- [ ] Dish detergent
- [ ] Facial tissues
- [ ] Unscented laundry detergent
- [ ] Light bulbs
- [ ] Paper plates
- [ ] Paper/plastic cups
- [ ] Paper towels
- [ ] Plastic utensils
- [ ] Stain remover
- [ ] Storage bags
- [ ] Toilet paper
- [ ] Trash bags
- [ ] _____
- [ ] _____
- [ ] _____
- [ ] _____
- [ ] _____
- [ ] _____
- [ ] _____

Personal Care

- ☐ Condoms
- ☐ Contact lens supplies
- ☐ Cotton swabs
- ☐ Nail files
- ☐ Heavy-flow sanitary napkins
- ☐ Shampoo, conditioner, and other hair-care products
- ☐ Shaving supplies
- ☐ Soap
- ☐ Witch hazel pads
- ☐ _____
- ☐ _____
- ☐ _____
- ☐ _____
- ☐ _____
- ☐ _____
- ☐ _____

Miscellaneous

- ☐ Envelopes
- ☐ Extra underwear and socks
- ☐ Pet supplies (such as food, litter, and heartworm and flea medications)
- ☐ Postage stamps
- ☐ _____
- ☐ _____
- ☐ _____
- ☐ _____
- ☐ _____
- ☐ _____
- ☐ _____

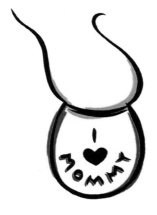

Duties to Divvy Up

It is realistic to assume that for at least the first six weeks after birth, you'll have no time or energy to focus on housekeeping. To help keep chores from building up, take some time in advance to determine who will be responsible for specific tasks after your baby is born. You can use the list below to help you get your thoughts in order. Put the designated person's initial in front of each task. Once the chores have been divvied up, post the list on the refrigerator or in some other central place where it will easily be noticed. Be explicit about what needs to be done, since not everyone defines "clean" the same way.

Daily

___ Drive other children to and
      from school and/or activities
___ Pick up clutter
___ Prepare breakfast
___ Prepare (or order) lunch
___ Prepare (or order) dinner
___ Wash dishes
___ Wipe down kitchen surfaces
___ Wash, fold, and put away laundry
___ Sort mail
___ Feed and take care of pets
___ _____
___ _____
___ _____

Weekly

___ Change bed sheets
___ Take out trash
___ Clean bathroom(s)
___ Clean kitchen
___ Shop for groceries
___ Take care of the yard
___ Dust
___ Sweep/vacuum floors
___ Drop off and pick up dry cleaning
___ Water plants
___ Clean cat box/birdcage/fish tank
___ _____
___ _____
___ _____

Monthly/Bimonthly/Periodically

__ Change washing machine lint trap
Dates to be done:

_____

__ Clean out refrigerator
Dates to be done:

_____

__ Have gutters cleaned
Dates to be done:

_____

__ Hose out garbage cans
Dates to be done:

_____

__ Refill prescriptions
Dates when next refills are due:

_____

__ Replace furnace filters
Dates to be done:

_____

__ Test smoke alarms
Dates to be done:

_____

__ Test carbon monoxide detectors
Dates to be done:

_____

__ Change oil and check filters and
fluid levels in car(s)
Points at which to be done:

_____

__ Prepare vehicle(s) for winter or summer
Dates to be done:

_____

__ Task: _____
Dates to be done:

_____

__ Task: _____
Dates to be done:

_____

__ Task: _____
Dates to be done:

_____

__ Task: _____
Dates to be done:

_____

__ Task: _____
Dates to be done:

_____

PART FOUR

Baby
Is Born

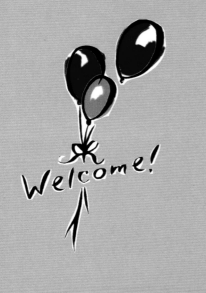

Welcome!

Baby Naming Tips

Picking a name for your baby can be one of the most entertaining of pregnancy pastimes. You may go through thousands of ideas before you find something that sounds right—and you may be shocked more than once by your partner's taste in names. If you and your partner haven't been able to arrive at a decision, try narrowing the possibilities down to your top ten favorites and go from there.

If your baby is on the way and you still can't decide, remember there's no law that you must name your child before you leave the healthcare facility (though you'll need to file the papers yourself, which is less convenient). Also, most states give you a year to change your baby's name without having to go through a formal legal procedure.

Here are some tips to keep in mind as you ponder your options.

❖ **Avoid misspellings of traditional names:** Your child will spend much of her life spelling out the name for others and correcting those who are confused. Studies have shown that kids with a "misspelled" name are often perceived as being less intelligent and are less likely to land job interviews when they grow up!

❖ **Beware of initials that spell out words:** Unless you want her schoolyard nickname to be "Dog," don't name your daughter Dawn Olsen Grant. Also remember that in traditional monograms, the initial for the surname appears in the middle, so Dawn Grant Olsen may be denied the pleasure of monogrammed luggage.

❖ **Remember nicknames:** If you can't stand "Liz," you probably shouldn't name your daughter Elizabeth. Nicknames are bestowed on the playground, and you'll have no control over them. Try to anticipate any unflattering variations that six-year-olds could come up with.

❖ **Check your name's popularity:** Your kid might like finding a key chain with her name on it every so often, but she will probably feel a little generic if five other kids in her class share her name, which could cause confusion and compel her to use a last initial.

Details, Details

This section will help you prepare for the day your baby arrives and the few months that follow. Obviously, you can't plan for everything, as childbirth has a way of following its own course. But taking care of some practical details ahead of time can be a huge help.

Toward that end, we've included space to write down the phone numbers of people to call when you go into labor, information about places offering takeout food or delivery near the birthing facility, and names and addresses for family and friends you intend to send birth announcements to. If you take time to compile this information in advance, you won't have to scramble when there are other pressing matters at hand.

Other useful sections you'll find in this chapter include space for tracking your contractions, a page to record details about baby after he arrives, and questions you might want to ask before you leave the hospital/birth center. And to help things go a little more smoothly once you're back home, there are some ready-made shopping lists along with a checklist of items to keep your diaper bag stocked with.

Contraction Chart

During the final month of your pregnancy, you may have more than one episode of contractions that make you wonder if it's really time to head to the birthing facility or if it's only a false alarm. Many women experience what's called prodromal labor before active labor starts. It's real labor, but it goes on for a while, sometimes weeks, without leading to cervical dilation. The difference between prodromal and active labor contractions is that the latter typically get consistently longer in duration, closer together, and stronger over the course of more than an hour or two.

If your contractions seem to be coming at a regular rate, time them by using a watch with a second hand, and record the information in the space provided below. When your contractions are regular for at least an hour and are getting stronger and more frequent, then it's probably time to call your care provider.

Time at start	Time at finish	Duration	Description

Time at start	Time at finish	Duration	Description

Important Numbers When Labor Starts

☐ Obstetrician's office:
　 Alternate number:
☐ Grandparents:

☐ Babysitter:
☐ Alternate babysitter:
☐ Labor assistant:

Other People to Call

☐ Name:
　 Phone:

☐ Name:
　 Phone:

☐ Name:
　 Phone:

☐ Name:
　 Phone:

☐ Name:
　 Phone:

☐ Name:
　 Phone:

☐ Name:
    Phone:

☐ Name:
    Phone:

☐ Name:
    Phone:

☐ Name:
    Phone:

☐ Name:
    Phone:

☐ Name:
    Phone:

☐ Name:
    Phone:

☐ Name:
    Phone:

☐ Name:
    Phone:

☐ Name:
    Phone:

☐ Name:
    Phone:

Takeout/Delivery

When you're at the hospital/birth center, it can be helpful to have information on nearby convenience stores, delis, and restaurants offering takeout and delivery. Fill in the information ahead of time so that your partner can refer to it when needed.

Name:

Phone:

Location:

Type of food:

Name:

Phone:

Location:

Type of food:

Name:

Phone:

Location:

Type of food:

Name:

Phone:

Location:

Type of food:

Name:

Phone:

Location:

Type of food:

Spreading the News

Use the following section to make note of those people to whom you want to send birth announcements. When an announcement has been sent, check the box next to the recipient's name to keep track.

☐ Name:
  Address:
  E-mail:

☐ Name:
  Address:
  E-mail:

☐ Name:
  Address:
  E-mail:

☐ Name:
  Address:
  E-mail:

☐ Name:
  Address:
  E-mail:

☐ Name:
  Address:
  E-mail:

☐ Name: _____
   Address: _____
   E-mail: _____

☐ Name: _____
   Address: _____
   E-mail: _____

☐ Name: _____
   Address: _____
   E-mail: _____

☐ Name: _____
   Address: _____
   E-mail: _____

☐ Name: _____
   Address: _____
   E-mail: _____

☐ Name: _____
   Address: _____
   E-mail: _____

☐ Name: _____
   Address: _____
   E-mail: _____

☐ Name: _____
   Address: _____
   E-mail: _____

☐ Name: _____
　　Address: _____
　　E-mail: _____

☐ Name: _____
　　Address: _____
　　E-mail: _____

☐ Name: _____
　　Address: _____
　　E-mail: _____

☐ Name: _____
　　Address: _____
　　E-mail: _____

☐ Name: _____
　　Address: _____
　　E-mail: _____

☐ Name: _____
　　Address: _____
　　E-mail: _____

☐ Name: _____
　　Address: _____
　　E-mail: _____

☐ Name: _____
　　Address: _____
　　E-mail: _____

All About Baby

❖ Full name: _____

❖ Why this name was chosen: _____
_____
_____

❖ Length of labor: _____

❖ Date and time of birth: _____

❖ Weight: _____

❖ Length: _____

❖ Apgar score: _____

❖ Baby looks the most like: _____

❖ Memories of our first moments as a new family: _____
_____
_____
_____
_____
_____
_____
_____
_____
_____
_____
_____
_____
_____
_____
_____
_____
_____
_____
_____
_____

Questions to Ask When Leaving the Hospital/Birth Center

Following are some questions you may want to ask.

❖ Is there a lactation consultant I can call if I have breastfeeding questions or issues? What's the number and the name of the contact person? _____

❖ How should I care for my stitches? _____

❖ Are there any activities I need to avoid, and if so, for how long? _____

_____

_____

❖ Are there any foods or medications I should avoid if I plan to breastfeed? _____

_____

_____

❖ Is there anything in particular I need to know about caring for my baby? _____

_____

_____

_____

❖ Can you give me pain medication to take home? _____
❖ Can I have a copy of any paperwork that I filled out? _____
❖ Will you be sending me an itemized bill? _____
❖ Other questions and notes: _____

_____

_____

_____

_____

After-Baby Shopping List

Once you're at home with your baby, you'll need not only your usual supplies and groceries but additional items just for the little one as well. When it's time to head to the store, use the handy shopping lists that follow to help make sure nothing is forgotten. Note the quantity, brand, and type so that whoever is running errands gets exactly what is needed. You can use the space at the end to write down any other items you want. For additional ideas, you may want to refer to the list of supplies on page 194. If you need more shopping lists, simply make photocopies of the ones provided here.

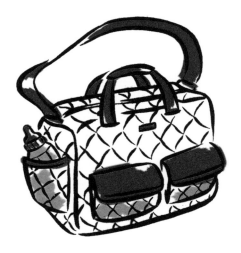

- [ ] Diapers
- [ ] Baby wipes
- [ ] Diaper rash ointment or powder
- [ ] Formula
- [ ] Bottles
- [ ] Nipples
- [ ] Pacifiers
- [ ] Mild, unscented laundry detergent
- [ ] Soap for you, guests, or baby
- [ ] Trash bags or refills for your diaper disposal system
- [ ] Paper towels
- [ ] Household cleaning products:

  - [ ] _____
  - [ ] _____
  - [ ] _____
  - [ ] _____

- [ ] Beverages for mom (especially if breastfeeding):

  - [ ] _____
  - [ ] _____
  - [ ] _____
  - [ ] _____

- [ ] Food for mom:

  - [ ] _____
  - [ ] _____
  - [ ] _____
  - [ ] _____
  - [ ] _____
  - [ ] _____

- [ ] Magazines or other reading material for mom:

  - [ ] _____
  - [ ] _____
  - [ ] _____
  - [ ] _____
  - [ ] _____
  - [ ] _____

- [ ] Anything else?

  - [ ] _____
  - [ ] _____
  - [ ] _____
  - [ ] _____
  - [ ] _____
  - [ ] _____
  - [ ] _____
  - [ ] _____
  - [ ] _____
  - [ ] _____
  - [ ] _____
  - [ ] _____

☐ Diapers _____

☐ Baby wipes _____

☐ Diaper rash ointment or powder _____

☐ Formula _____

☐ Bottles _____

☐ Nipples _____

☐ Pacifiers _____

☐ Mild, unscented laundry detergent _____

☐ Soap for you, guests, or baby _____

☐ Trash bags or refills for your diaper disposal system _____

☐ Paper towels _____

☐ Household cleaning products:

   ☐ _____ ☐ _____

   ☐ _____ ☐ _____

☐ Beverages for mom (especially if breastfeeding):

   ☐ _____ ☐ _____

   ☐ _____ ☐ _____

☐ Food for mom:

   ☐ _____ ☐ _____

   ☐ _____ ☐ _____

   ☐ _____ ☐ _____

☐ Magazines or other reading material for mom:

   ☐ _____ ☐ _____

   ☐ _____ ☐ _____

   ☐ _____ ☐ _____

☐ Anything else?

   ☐ _____ ☐ _____

   ☐ _____ ☐ _____

   ☐ _____ ☐ _____

   ☐ _____ ☐ _____

   ☐ _____ ☐ _____

   ☐ _____ ☐ _____

☐ Diapers

☐ Baby wipes

☐ Diaper rash ointment or powder

☐ Formula

☐ Bottles

☐ Nipples

☐ Pacifiers

☐ Mild, unscented laundry detergent

☐ Soap for you, guests, or baby

☐ Trash bags or refills for your diaper disposal system

☐ Paper towels

☐ Household cleaning products:

    ☐ _____   ☐ _____

    ☐ _____   ☐ _____

☐ Beverages for mom (especially if breastfeeding):

    ☐ _____   ☐ _____

    ☐ _____   ☐ _____

☐ Food for mom:

    ☐ _____   ☐ _____

    ☐ _____   ☐ _____

    ☐ _____   ☐ _____

☐ Magazines or other reading material for mom:

    ☐ _____   ☐ _____

    ☐ _____   ☐ _____

    ☐ _____   ☐ _____

☐ Anything else?

    ☐ _____   ☐ _____

    ☐ _____   ☐ _____

    ☐ _____   ☐ _____

    ☐ _____   ☐ _____

    ☐ _____   ☐ _____

    ☐ _____   ☐ _____

What's in a Diaper Bag?

If you haven't known many babies, you may be wondering what's in a diaper bag besides diapers. Following is a list of what you may wish to pack when you leave the house with your baby. Note that it's a good idea to keep your diaper bag stocked and by your front door in case you need to leave the house in a hurry. Also, if you drive, it can be helpful to have a backup supply of essentials in your car.

- ☐ Diapers (two or three minimum)
- ☐ Portable changing pad or a small towel (something to protect baby's bottom from surfaces and vice versa)
- ☐ Pre-moistened baby wipes (use travel-size packages, or carry individual wipes in a plastic sandwich bag that seals shut)
- ☐ Diaper rash ointment, if baby has a rash
- ☐ Plastic bag to hold any dirty clothes until you get home
- ☐ Change of clothes for baby
- ☐ Tissues, washcloth, or cloth diaper in case you encounter spit-up or a leaky diaper
- ☐ If bottle-feeding:
    - ☐ bottle
    - ☐ nipple
    - ☐ nipple ring
    - ☐ pre-measured powdered formula
    - ☐ bottled water for mixing
- ☐ Spare nursing pads, if you're breastfeeding or still lactating
- ☐ Seasonal outerwear for baby (hat in summer; jacket, blanket, or bunting in winter)
- ☐ Sunscreen for you and your baby if you're going to be outside
- ☐ Pacifiers, if your baby uses them
- ☐ Antibacterial hand gel for yourself

PART FIVE

Personal

Directory

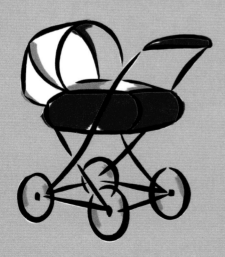

Diaper-Changing Basics

If you've never changed a diaper before, the task can be intimidating. Here are the basics when using disposables.

- ❖ Prepare what you'll need first:
  - Remove a new diaper from the package; unfold and place it next to you on the changing table.
  - Have pre-moistened baby wipes or a warm, damp washcloth ready.
  - Make sure there's a garbage bag in the diaper pail.
- ❖ Lay the baby on his back on a changing pad or towel, being sure to support his head and neck at all times.
- ❖ Remove the old diaper. If it has Velcro® brand tabs, you can roll it up from back to front and use the tabs to make a tidy package.
- ❖ Remove dirty clothes if the diaper has leaked, and launder them as soon as possible.
- ❖ Clean off the baby with the wipes or damp washcloth, being sure to go from front to back to keep all fecal material away from the urinary tract area.
- ❖ If it looks like it's going to take more than a few wipes to clean the baby, and the umbilical cord and circumcision sites have healed, consider giving the baby a "bottom bath" in the sink with a washcloth.
- ❖ After the baby is clean and dry, lift up his rump by holding his ankles up with one hand, and then slide the new diaper under the baby's bottom with your other hand. (Most diapers have a design on the front of the waistband to indicate which part is the front.)
- ❖ Apply kaolin clay powder, cornstarch-based powder, or diaper rash ointment if baby's bottom looks red.
- ❖ Peel off the tabs that cover the tape or unfold the Velcro® brand strips, and pull the diaper firmly around baby so that it will stay on. Press the tabs into the soft part of the front of the diaper.

Voilà!

Important Contacts & Directions

This directory has been provided so that you can keep all your pregnancy-related contact information—from that of your care provider to your doula—in one place. Also included are spaces to fill in the phone numbers of people who provide other services that you depend on, such as your plumber and electrician, so that once baby has arrived and you're busy attending to her needs, your partner, friends, and family will be better able to take care of household maintenance. In addition, there's a handy chart for filling in the names, numbers, and e-mail addresses of people in your childbirth class so that you can keep in touch with them. And, last but not least, there's a place for you to write down directions to the birthing facility.

Accountant

Name:

Address:

Phone:

Fax: E-mail:

Auto Mechanic

Name:

Address:

Phone:

Fax:

Babysitters

Name:

Address:

Phone:

Name:

Address:

Phone:

Name: _____

Address: _____

Phone: _____

Name: _____

Address: _____

Phone: _____

Bank

Name: _____

Address: _____

Phone: _____

Building Superintendent

Name: _____

Address: _____

Phone: _____

Fax: _____ E-mail: _____

Childbirth Educator

Name: _____

Class address: _____

Phone: _____

Fax: _____ E-mail: _____

Cleaning Service

Name: _____

Address: _____

Phone: _____

Fax: _____ E-mail: _____

Computer Technician
Name:

Address:

Phone:

Fax: E-mail:

Dentists
Name:

Address:

Phone:

Fax:

Name:

Address:

Phone:

Fax:

Dry Cleaner
Name:

Address:

Phone:

Electrician
Name:

Address:

Phone:

Fax:

Handyman
Name:

Address:

Phone:

Fax:

Health Insurance Company
Name:

Address:

Phone:

Policy number:

Hospital/Birth Center
Name:

Address:

Phone (main number):

    (obstetrics ward):

Fax:

Kennel
Name:

Address:

Phone:

Fax:

Labor Assistant
Name:

Address:

Phone:

Fax:

Lactation Consultant

Name:

Address:

Phone:

Fax:

Landlord

Name:

Address:

Phone:

Fax:

Midwife

Name:

Address:

Phone:

Fax:

Mortgage Company

Name:

Address:

Phone:

Fax:

Neighbors

Name:

Address:

Phone:

Name:

Address:

Phone:

Name:

Address:

Phone:

Name:

Address:

Phone:

Name:

Address:

Phone:

Obstetrician

Name:

Address:

Phone:

Fax:

Pediatrician

Name:

Address:

Phone:

Fax:

Pharmacy

Name:

Address:

Phone:

Fax:

Plumber

Name:

Address:

Phone:

Fax:

Psychiatrist

Name:

Address:

Phone:

Fax:

Taxi Services

Company name:

Phone:

Company name:

Phone:

Veterinarian

Name:

Address:

Phone:

Fax:

Yard Service

Name:

Address:

Phone:

Fax:

My Childbirth Class Contact List

Name	Phone #	E-mail

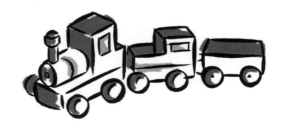

Getting to the Hospital/Birth Center

Number to call for a ride to the hospital/birth center when I go into labor:

Number for alternate driver or cab company: _____

Directions: _____

_____

_____

_____

_____

_____

_____

_____

_____

_____

_____

_____

_____

Alternate route: _____

_____

_____

_____

_____

_____

_____

_____

_____

_____

_____

_____

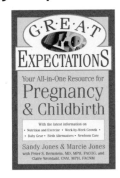